# The Hearing Impaired Child

# The Hearing Impaired Child

Dan Goldstein

NFER-NELSON

Published by The NFER-NELSON Publishing Company Ltd.,
Darville House, 2 Oxford Road East,
Windsor, Berkshire SL4 1DF, England.

First published 1989
© 1989, Dan Goldstein

Typeset by David John Services Ltd., Slough
Printed by Billing & Sons Ltd, Worcester

ISBN 0 7005 1243 8

Code 8334 02 4

# Contents

# List of Figures and Tables

# Acknowledgements

My grateful thanks to all the children who have been an inspiration. Also to my colleagues who have helped me, over the years, to further my understanding.

# Foreword

On the day his elevation to the peerage was announced, Lewis Silkin sat with his wife in the restaurant of an hotel in Cornwall. It was a modest place, but one with aspirations. The waiters, who all seemed to be Spanish, were busily serving the five-course set meal. For some reason, never explained, the waiters did not go near Lord Silkin, no matter how hard he tried to gain attention. After about 45 minutes, when most of the diners were well advanced with their meals, he leaned across. Very mildly in the circumstances and with the careful analysis that was his hallmark as a solicitor, he said, 'It is seldom that one has the opportunity of speaking in absolute terms. I think on this occasion, I can honestly say, without fear of contradiction, that this is the worst service I have ever had.'

Some of the topics dealt with in this book, for all their seeming blandness, give rise to heated controversies. Every attempt will be made to treat them in the most even-handed way possible, but there is no way each statement can be qualified with Lord Silkin's exactitude. A wide range of individuals will be described. Of necessity they will be grouped for the purposes of making general statements. There will inevitably be exceptions to the rule. The same is true of certain techniques referred to. They hold good for the majority of cases alluded to. But there are sure to be some who will maintain a contrary view. The reader is asked to bear this constantly in mind.

# 1 Introduction

## Statutory considerations

This book is primarily intended to give non-specialist teachers an understanding of different types of hearing loss, how they are diagnosed and what teaching approaches are useful. The recommendations made take into account recent legislation and the imminent introduction of the national curriculum. It is important to bear in mind the fact that, 'The Secretary of State believes that all pupils, including those with special educational needs, should have the opportunity to obtain the maximum benefit possible from it'. As 'the 1981 Act placed LEAs under a duty to secure that, subject to conditions specified in Section 2(3), children with statements should be educated in ordinary schools' (Draft Circular [–/89] Revision of Circular 1/83), there has been pressure for more disabled children to be in mainstream settings.

There is provision for disapplication of the National Curriculum in certain cases. From what has been published to date it would appear that the primary reasons for exempting children for up to six months is to allow for the effects of illness to be overcome or enough time to become proficient in English in the case of children for whom it is a second language. But as far as children with special educational needs are concerned teachers must anticipate teaching within the framework of the national curriculum, even though as the proposals for English point out, 'some may hover around the level 1 attainments for the whole of their school careers' (p. 59; 13.4).

## Incidence of hearing impairment

Serious hearing loss occurs in about two per thousand of the population, the same sort of incidence as for other major disabilities. Apart from these cases it has been estimated that as many as 50 per cent of inner-city children under the age of seven may have transient hearing losses and up to 10 per cent a recurrent or persistent loss sufficient to affect educational progress. Given numbers of this order it is unlikely that a teacher will never be faced with a hearing impaired child. A loss of sufficient magnitude to make communication difficult is less likely to be encountered. When it is, it might be because parents insist on mainstream provision, a partially hearing unit is housed in the school and children from the partially hearing unit are integrated in mainstream classes for part of their timetable, or there is no local specialized provision of any kind and a boarding school is the only alternative to the neighbourhood school.

## Qualifications required to teach hearing impaired children

At present special qualifications are mandatory to teach both 'deaf' and 'blind' children, so it is quite natural for a teacher without such qualifications to feel apprehensive when confronted with a child who has either one or possibly a combination of the two disabilities to some degree. It is possible for teachers without prior qualifications to teach hearing impaired children, but it should only be under the supervision of a qualified teacher and be accompanied by a recognized in-service training course leading to a specialist qualification. It is hoped that what follows will help the ordinary classroom teacher to understand more about hearing losses and of equal importance how they may teach more effectively. Any teacher with experience of hearing impaired children, including specialists, knows that there are limitations as to what can be achieved. The aim of this book is to encourage all teachers to assist hearing impaired children realize their fullest potential, while accepting it may not be possible for them to attain quite the same standards as children with normal hearing. Some idea of why this should be so is contained in Chapter 7 on language and emotional development.

## Terms commonly used in reports

To set the scene for what is meant by *hearing impairment* a number of commonly used terms will be introduced. These, together with data presented in the other chapters will clarify information contained in reports included in the child's records. Hearing impairment is an umbrella term, requiring more precise definition if it is to be meaningful in respect of a particular child. Basically there are four parameters: *age of onset; cause; degree and type.* The *age of onset* is important because impairment after speech and language have been acquired leads to less marked effects than when it is congenital or occurs very early in life. Hearing can of course be impaired or lost at any age. Present estimates of *causes* are that 60 per cent of *severe* and *profound congenital hearing losses* are due to otherwise fit and healthy parents both having a recessive gene which leads to deafness in their offspring. Apart from the hearing loss the children are usually healthy.

Practice varies considerably from area to area in terms of what information is made available to the class teacher. When the only reports on a child's hearing difficulties are locked away with medical records, a peripatetic teacher of the hearing impaired may be able to supply the relevant facts – in the event of their not being made available by the school doctor or nurse. The term 'hearing impaired', already employed a number of times, is now used instead of deaf because even 'deaf' individuals can usually hear some sounds. Unfortunately the new term obscures the *degree* of loss. Various types of hearing impairment and hearing losses are described later.

Confusion can be caused because *hearing loss* and hearing impairment are often used interchangeably. When a loss is congenital the degree of hearing impairment should be specified. In practice reference is made to the size of the loss even though better levels of hearing have never existed. The point to remember is that what is said in reports refers to the situation at the time of the tests. With certain kinds of hearing loss, especially if they are amenable to treatment, there could be an improvement. In other cases a steady deterioration might ensue. The incidence of sudden loss is rare, but when it does occur the impact is quite shattering for the individual concerned.

The amount or degree of hearing loss ranges from profound, through *moderate* to *mild.* The profound or virtually total inability to hear is what most people think of as deaf. The advent of special services for the deaf on television has tended to reinforce this notion, suggesting that the principal form of communication for the deaf is through the use of signs and finger spelling. As it happens only a small percentage of all hearing impaired people rely wholly on these methods of communication. At the other end of the range mild hearing impairment is quite slight and likely to become familiar to most people as they get older. When hearing fails due to age a hearing aid can be useful. Just how useful may be gauged by the frequency and length of time it is worn. Many of the aids issued to elderly people languish unused in drawers, a fact explained away by reference to age, cantankerousness, an unwillingness to make an effort, or the loss of interest generally. Yet glasses, which are just as much of a nuisance are worn. The difference is glasses correct slight visual defects more or less completely. Hearing aids are not so precise in their function. This is dealt with in greater detail later. It has been mentioned at this point because the limitations of hearing aids, despite the enormous benefits they can confer, are still imperfect instruments. The wearing of them does not automatically solve all the hearing problems of users, a point that cannot be made too often.

A mild hearing loss is a bit of a nuisance to older people. Much of the time they do not have too great a problem, though they may tend to accuse others of mumbling. Noisy conditions present greater difficulties both for them and the greater losses about to be described. Moderate hearing losses entail missing much more of what is said and many everyday sounds are often not heard, for example the doorbell or the telephone. Once this degree of loss is encountered a hearing aid becomes a necessity, though in quiet surroundings, providing interlocutors speak up clearly, conversation can still be followed. Severe hearing loss removes the ability to make sense of what is heard unless some additional clues, such as lip reading, are used. A profound hearing loss is a major disability that affects the individual's ability to communicate. It not only prevents those affected from hearing what is said it mars the quality of their own speech. This can make it somewhat difficult for those to whom they speak to understand. The vicious circle that ends in isolation starts at this point.

## Origins of special education

The development of provisions to educate the hearing impaired has a long history, starting with the Romans, if not earlier. Renewed interest was shown in Europe in the 16th century and institutions were set up to educate the profoundly deaf. By and large they were taught separately by very specialized methods. An overview is given in Appendix A. The last century saw a further upsurge of interest in the education of the 'deaf' and 'blind', which led to the enactment of a statute making special qualifications for teachers of the deaf and the blind mandatory in Britain. Other European countries took similar measures. More special schools were set up. Many of these were residential and some such as the Royal School for the Deaf in Manchester and the Royal Victoria school for the Deaf in Margate still function. These catered for those whose hearing losses were evidently so great as to prevent them from learning speech and language normally through hearing. Some children with moderate hearing losses suffered the fate of being considered mentally defective or at a later date, educationally subnormal. 'Moderate learning difficulty' is the current terminology.

## Effects of hearing impairment in the classroom

Hearing impaired children's slowness in learning is still being put down to a general lack of ability rather than the effects of hearing difficulties. I came across a case recently when I was asked to assess a child's special educational needs. It was thought by her own teacher and the headteacher who had observed her, that she might be better off in a special school on account of her learning difficulties. Her mother and the Head of the school, both present during the assessment, were surprised by the quality of some of her answers. Indeed overall she showed herself to be well within the normal range of abilities. A quick and simple test (see page 120) showed she had a significant hearing loss. This was confirmed later under clinical conditions and since it was a curable condition, arrangements were made for surgical treatment. After the operation she was reported to be still slow. After years of not hearing properly it is inevitable that bringing her hearing to within normal limits would not effect a magical transformation. 'But if she can now hear normally, why isn't she responding normally?' is a typical question, also asked when children are fitted with aids. Just because the brain is locked away in a bony skull does not make it different in essence from any other part of the body in terms of basic function. No one would expect to run a marathon without a lot of intensive training beforehand. The skills and stamina have to be built up over time. If it takes so long just to get comparatively simple muscles into shape, it is obviously going to take a lot longer when it comes to extremely complex intellectual functions.

Apart from children in the same position as the one just described, there are others whose lives have been transformed by the advent of hearing aids. By wearing them consistently many are able to cope in a normal school setting. In effect children with moderate to severe losses are enabled to learn in a way that was only true for those with quite mild losses – always provided optimal conditions are made available. About that more anon. Even so some children in this category need the extra support provided by a partially hearing unit, or at least some additional, specialized teaching input.

## Issues

There are contentious educational issues which are peculiar to the hearing impaired, others apply with equal force to most disabilities. Some will only be mentioned in the introduction and not referred to again, leaving the remainder for more detailed discussion in later chapters. It will be appreciated that in a book of this size it is impossible to cover each and every area of importance in depth, so the aim is to give essential information and provide a feel for the issues involved. There is no typical hearing impaired child who can be described to personify the rest. As will become clear, hearing impaired children have to be considered very much more as individuals, taking due note of local influences.

## Present educational provision for the hearing impaired

### *Pre-school*

The way education is currently provided for the hearing impaired is a bone of contention. Before explaining why, the various specialists who are likely to come into contact with hearing impaired children will be listed. Who is available varies throughout the country. All local education authorities have a peripatetic service for the hearing impaired, staff by peripatetic teachers of the hearing impaired with an additional teaching qualification in respect of the hearing impaired. Prior to taking up such work the teachers will have had experience in one or more sort of specialized educational setting for the hearing impaired. Many have a Diploma in Audiology, so that in all two extra years of full-time training have been completed after initial qualification, usually with punctuation to gain more teaching experience as a specialist between times. Their first contact with a local hearing impaired child may be in an audiology clinic. Such clinics do not exist in all parts of the country. Some families have to make long treks to a specialist hospital department. In the event of a hearing loss being confirmed many further visits are bound to follow. These are very demanding, especially if a strict appointment system is not adhered to. Difficult journeys, followed by long waits can be very daunting, especially if there are other children in tow. In such circumstances, FTA (failed to attend) occasionally written on hospital records is not surprising. If it happens more than once or twice the parent is branded as uncooperative.

If there has been any reason to suspect a hearing loss or parents have been suspicious all is not well, the results obtained in an audiology clinic may simply confirm fears and expectations, quantifying the nature and degree of a hearing loss. Even when this is the case, it is still very traumatic for the parents. For parents for whom the revelation is wholly unexpected or denied, albeit subconsciously, their distress can be quite devastating initially. A child welcomed and regarded at birth as normal is exposed as invisibly damaged. So apart from the usual reactions to discovering an infant has a hearing loss there are additional stresses. On top of all this they have to cope with the various support agencies who become involved: ENT consultant; audiological physician; paediatrician; physiological measurement technician; peripatetic teacher of the hearing impaired; genetic counsellor; health visitor and social worker. The physiological measurement technician often carries out routine hearing tests and makes ear moulds, in addition to a wide range of other functions. At least five of these specialists will be involved if a hearing aid is issued, the whole lot in some cases.

The peripatetic teacher of the hearing impaired gives guidance and support to the parents and/or any other regular caretaker in addition to advising on the use of any hearing aid issued. Examples of the suggestions made are set out in later chapters. The important practices that have to be observed are that if an aid is needed it is kept in good working order and it is worn consistently throughout the day. Activities to enhance awareness of as many environmental sounds as possible are used. Sound-making toys and a variety of musical instruments, especially the percussive ones, are employed in play situations into which elements of direction can be introduced. This stimulates a basic interaction between what is heard and what is done. It is at a lower level than obeying spoken instructions, but it has the same fundamental characteristic of linking hearing and doing. Naturally every opportunity is taken to draw attention to and encourage communication through spoken language.

## School-age provision

A variety of educational establishments exist to make what is considered to be the best provision for hearing impaired children. In some instances children start in the nursery class of a special school as young as two years of age. Apart from day schools there are also residential schools catering for children with profound hearing losses. Of the latter type one is a grammar school, namely Mary Hare. Other schools, both day and residential, have pupils with the usual range of intelligence. Some of these have special units as well, for children with additional disabilities, e.g. The Royal Victoria School for the Deaf with its Deaf/Blind Unit, and another for children with behavioural and emotional difficulties. Some schools take partially hearing children, who can learn mainly through hearing. Day special schools usually only have profoundly hearing impaired children of normal intellectual ability. When other problems arise arrangements are often made for them to transfer to a residential school. If a pre-school child goes to one of these full-time special schools the peripatetic teacher of the hearing impaired no longer has any dealings with the child since the teachers will all have comparable specialist qualifications. Contact continues with children who go to day nurseries and later to ordinary schools. The level of staffing in any given peripatetic service determines the amount of direct teaching given. When working for one authority as a peripatetic teacher of the hearing impaired I was able to see pre-school, nursery and infant children for about an hour, two or three times a week. With another, due to poorer staffing ratios, it was almost impossible to manage once a fortnight. So it is very unlikely any child in primary school will be taught on a regular basis. Once children are at secondary school the peripatetic teacher of the hearing impaired will do little more than check to see all members of staff are aware of the presence of a hearing impaired child, providing generalized guide-lines and saying who to contact for hearing aid maintenance.

In addition to special schools there are units. One London school has a unit for children with profound hearing losses. The children with normal hearing have become so expert at signing that they have completely undermined the whole purpose of integration since they omit to speak to the hearing impaired children when signing. Children with all their faculties are very adaptable and unconsciously alter the level at which they pitch their language when addressing those younger than themselves. In the setting cited, the hearing children, knowing what they say cannot be heard, do not make any unnecessary efforts, adapting their behaviour to suit the circumstances in a similar way. Apart from the children receiving special education there are large numbers with varying degrees of hearing loss scattered through day nurseries and schools. Most will only have mild or moderate losses, others quite severe ones. How successful they are depends on the usual range of factors: the innate ability of the child; the amount of help and support provided by the home; how much extra help is available within the school, etc. Each case must be judged according to individual circumstances. Blanket prescriptions should not be made on the basis of isolated cases.

Whatever educational provision is arranged for a hearing impaired child : special school; partially hearing unit; mainstream with support or simply monitoring by a peripatetic teacher of the hearing impaired, the emphasis always has to be on the development of communication skills. In special schools the approaches used tend to be more formal than in many others. This is necessary for the children to acquire the skills needed to understand what is said to them and speak to others in an intelligible way. Some never achieve either to any great degree. Most children in partially hearing units can hold conversations, though this is not invariably so. Again it is a question of terminology. One parent refused to consider a recommendation for a special school and indeed moved to an area where a partially hearing unit was the designated provision. In that particular instance the class so designated contained a mixture of children with losses ranging from moderate to profound. Furthermore there was no integration for any of the pupils. Another parent whose son was in an ordinary school became very upset and tearful when a partially hearing unit was suggested for the umpteenth time. She only agreed to visit one when it was put to her that I would be failing to fulfil professional responsibilities if what was considered to be the most appropriate advice were not given. The partially hearing unit in question consisted of several classes, housed in a mainstream school. Some of the pupils spent hardly any time in the partially hearing unit, having attained requisite standards to function well with very little additional support. When we next met after her visit I was practically accused of having failed to tell her of this wonderful provision. Then she arranged for the transfer of the twin brother to the same school and upset the headteacher of the first school into the bargain.

Sometimes hearing impaired children who have coped in an ordinary primary school with peripatetic support and perhaps additional teaching provided via the statementing procedure need to go to a secondary school in which a partially hearing unit is housed. Similarly, though more rarely, a child will transfer from a primary partially hearing unit to a school for children with profound hearing losses. Whether such a pattern will continue once the programmes of study for the national curriculum are fully operational, remains to be seen. They should result in a greater uniformity at all stages, from 5 to 16. In theory programmes suitably modified for children with special educational needs will be published, along with appropriate standardized assessment tasks. If practice matches rhetoric, the structures should make it easier to provide adequately for children with mild to moderate hearing losses and in some cases of moderate to severe losses. As losses become greater, the ability to benefit from mainstream provision becomes more and more dependent on higher intellectual ability and what appears to be a greater innate facility for acquiring verbal language in some hearing impaired children than in others.

## Educational approaches

There are two principal educational approaches used to educate the hearing impaired with severe or profound losses. This is reflected in the personal philosophies of peripatetic teachers of the hearing impaired and school based teachers. Some are what may be termed 'pure oralists'. They believe all hearing impaired children must be taught through speech and lip reading, making the fullest possible use of any residual hearing, without any form of signs or gestures. The most extreme proponents of this approach have been known to tell parents to sit on their hands rather than make any sign or gesture, thereby ignoring normal body language and the way in which it is used to convey information. There are others who subscribe to 'Total Communication' for children with very great hearing losses. The same amount of attention is paid to the use of residual hearing, speech and lip reading, but in addition natural gestures are used as well as signs of the sort used on television. Deaf adults tend to favour *Total Communication*. It permits communication at an earlier age than when relying wholly on speech. If the parents of the child are deaf and use sign language themselves then they will teach their child to do likewise, no matter what is recommended by the peripatetic teacher of the hearing impaired. The same is likely to be true of their reactions to audiological physicians and some ENT consultants, especially those trained at Manchester – since they more than others have tended to espouse the pure oral approach. The situation is rather different for parents with no prior experience of hearing loss in children. They consult those whom they believe to be experts and quite naturally do as they are advised. I have met parents, who having initially embraced the oral approach whole-heartedly, later expressed regret that they had not been informed of other options earlier.

Before passing on brief mention must be made about other methods of teaching that surface in different guises from time to time. Finger spelling may be used to indicate every letter. In effect this is a straightforward transformation of print into hand movements. It is many years since I have encountered this being practised as a whole school policy. It was very useful with one very deaf boy who had autistic features and would not look directly at anyone. Since finger spelling and signing could be employed in front of his lowered level of gaze it provided the earliest means of teaching. *Cued speech* is a variant of finger spelling. In this case it is speech sounds that are indicated by hand configurations and movements, which means there are more than the 26 associated with finger spelling. The aim of cued speech is to help differentiate between sounds that have almost identical visual patterns, e.g. k/g; t/d; m/b, etc. It can only be used in conjunction with speech. Then there is *acupedia*. This entails relying totally on hearing. No visual clues are permitted at all. The theory is that by making use of amplified sound any residual hearing can be used to teach the child to understand the spoken word and to speak. Claims for success have been made in a very small number of cases.

Approaches to a different kind of problem are instructive. In Chailey Heritage a lot of work was done to make mobile limbs for children who suffered from the effects of thalidomide. The joints were made to move by compressed air. Some limbless children were enabled, amidst a great deal of hissing, to take faltering steps. A man who adopted one such disabled child thought that this was ridiculous and designed the Chailey Chariot, a wheeled vehicle that permitted the child to move around freely and adjust to different heights suited to immediate needs. There is still a domineering attitude of many able bodied people that anyone without comparable abilities must be made normal. It is argued here that the most important need is to value the individual and help him or her to achieve the fullest and richest lifestyle by whatever means are most suitable in his or her case. This will never be possible if preconceived notions are clung to, come hell or high water, as has been done by some practitioners of one persuasion or another.

## Integration

All the issues surrounding integration will not be dealt with at length, but some reference to them must be made. In the normal course of development most children cannot say much before the age of 1 to $1^1/2$ years of age. A lot of language has already been learned however. When the necessary intellectual and articulatory skills have been acquired it is simply a question of putting into practice what is already known. Much of what is known has been learned incidentally. For hearing impaired children to learn to lip read and communicate through speech, a much more deliberate effort has been made. They are not ready to make such efforts before about the age of $1^1/2$, even though babies will mimic facial expressions from as young as ten days of age and learn from observation a wide variety of signs and gestures. Some of these are clearly iconographic: beckoning towards, waving away; pretending to eat, and so on. So communication *per se* is established. Ideas are formed and provide the basis for the understanding later given expression by speech and verbal language. That was a point regularly made by the Headmaster of a special school when parents commented upon the quality of the hearing impaired children's speech. First it is necessary to give them something to talk about. In the majority of cases, once they were able to formulate sequences of grammatically correct sentences, speech improved markedly. The teaching of speech always went alongside everything else that was taught, in order to provide practice in the relevant skills. Often these were not fully utilized until after leaving school. Then, when there had been the everyday pressures to communicate as clearly as possible, the by then young adults, drew upon their own resources to effect self-improvement. Surely it could be argued, if they had been integrated that pressure would have occurred earlier with concomitant benefits? That would be true provided the teaching ratio remains the same (that is, one teacher for every eight pupils) and speech and language teaching forms an integral part of each and every lesson, in addition to individual speech teaching.

In my experience profoundly hearing impaired children, with profoundly hearing impaired parents who use signs, often develop a better grasp of language at an earlier age than other profoundly hearing impaired children, whose parents do not know how to communicate with them from birth. A seven-year-old child I taught when working in a residential school for the deaf wrote in a weekly letter home, 'Dear mummy, please thank aunty Betty for her nice letter and tell her I have been too busy to write.' Given her age the ability to formulate such thoughts was good in itself. Committing them to paper represents an acceptable level of attainment for that age, but then there is a great deal of emphasis on writing from an early stage in schools for the hearing impaired.

The curriculum of the hearing impaired has of necessity to be much more carefully structured and internally integrated than for children with normal hearing. This is in order to present repeatedly, in as many settings as possible, any new words and grammatical constructions encountered. Unless this is done there is insufficient exposure for them to be remembered and incorporated by hearing impaired children in their own usage. The repetitions serve to reinforce what has been learned as well as providing the opportunities for checking on correct understanding. Furthermore it assists in forming more generalized associations, something the hearing impaired often have difficulties with. The implications of these brief statements will be appreciated more fully within Chapter 4. To fulfil these requirements adequately calls for a lot more time and effort than when teaching other children, hence the small classes in special schools and partially hearing units. Naturally when a child is one of a class of 30 the same detailed attention cannot be given as to one of six or eight. A hearing loss is a full-time disability, therefore it calls for full-time educational provision, whatever the setting in which it is given.

The Warnock Report set out a particular point of view in respect of integration and the 1981 Education Act incorporated many of its recommendations. Together they created a climate that led parents to expect a free choice as to which school their child should attend. By some this has been interpreted as meaning all children should be educated in a mainstream setting. Grievances reported in the press publicise cases where expectations have not been met. Because the Report and the Act generated a great deal of discussion about integration, most readers are likely to have well-articulated views on the subject of whether all children with disabilities should be integrated. Those who are for will ignore any arguments to the contrary – unless some direct, personal experience persuades them otherwise. Those who are opposed, and these are currently likely to be few in number, need no convincing. Any waverers in respect of the hearing impaired may reach their own conclusions from the information given in this book, without further advocacy or special pleading. When considering the pros and cons of integration the reader is asked to make a clear mental distinction between being in the presence of and being in the company of. The latter entails full-blooded participation on the basis of equal standing. I was told by a Director of Special Education in Stockholm, that no special educational establishments exist there. This statement was then qualified by mention of all the additional input provided within a mainstream setting. Does a child so identified and so encumbered by individual attention meet the criterion for being in the company of his or her peers? In the United States of America there is legislation that refers to 'the least restrictive environment'. Carol Amon, a Consultant in Colarado has posed the question, 'What about value differences relating to the need to interact with hearing impaired peers?' Her contribution and that of others in Auditory Disorders in School Children (2nd ed) set out in more detail many of the reservations I express in the course of this book. This is mentioned because at the final draft stage of this book an editorial enquiry suggested that some of the more negative aspects should be toned down. By chance I had been asked to review the American book and the views expressed quite independently in relation to a very different educational setting were very familiar from my own experiences in this country.

From the foregoing it will be clear that there are many factors which serve to create a kaleidoscopic range of interactions. Exactly what provision is made for any specific child takes on the nature of a lottery, depending on: the parental reaction to the hearing loss; place of residence; the prejudices of the professionals with whom the parents come into contact when a hearing loss is first diagnosed; whether he or she gets caught up in some form of experimental provisions and what resources are available locally.

The information contained in the remainder of this book will certainly not provide all the answers when it comes to teaching hearing impaired children in mainstream settings. It should help teachers to formulate questions that open up avenues as to how the teaching of hearing impaired children may be made most effective. Perhaps when considering the teacher/learner relationship, the commonplace questions: *Who* does *what, when, where, how* and *why?* can form a useful starting point. In the event of doubt they can provide the framework for evaluation, both in respect of what is being learned and what is being taught. With hearing impaired children it is likely these questions will need to be asked frequently. As regards what is taught, the national curriculum will largely take care of that. It will also provide a ready frame of reference for making comparisons between the attainments of hearing impaired children and expected norms, by means of ongoing assessments and Standardized Assessment Tasks. That leaves the teacher with the question how. Much of what follows is addressed to answering that question.

# 2 Causes of Hearing Loss

In the introduction a genetic defect was mentioned as a common cause of profound hearing loss and the likelihood of those so affected being otherwise healthy. This is certainly not the case when the cause is maternal rubella. Depending on when the infection occurred, the results can be disastrous. Early infection, when the central nervous system is developing, damages ears, eyes, heart, digestive system and motor control. All this is often accompanied by gross intellectual retardation. Therefore the immunization of girls against Rubella is always to be recommended. If there is total compliance it is hoped that Rubella may be eradicated in the same way as smallpox. Other viral infections can affect hearing at any time in life, for example mumps, measles and meningitis. Meningitis may lead to damage to the central nervous system, so that in addition to a hearing loss learning difficulties and personality changes arise.

A very common cause of hearing loss is *otitis media*. One variant of it is called *glue ear*. This is never so severe as the most extreme form of loss arising from other causes, but might none the less have a quite significant effect on a child's ability to learn. (More details are given in the Glossary.) Since it affects young children at a time when the most rapid language development is taking place it should never be overlooked, even though if left untreated it will in most cases clear up spontaneously by the time a child is nearing the end of the primary stage at the latest. This is due to structural changes which occur with growth improving the drainage of the middle ear. There are a whole host of other causes of congenital hearing impairment, but since many are rarities they are not listed here. For anyone interested reference can be made to a handbook of audiology, though this is not to be recommended to the squeamish.

The remainder of this chapter is presented in five sections:

## The ear

The structure of the ear, how sound is conducted from the outside world and transformed into nervous impulses are described, highlighting features of importance in an educational setting. There has been recent research which could go some way towards explaining why hearing losses regarded as insignificant by doctors should be dealt with much more seriously by teachers.

## Hearing tests

Although classroom teachers are never likely to be involved in the giving of a hearing test, the careful way in which they are conducted exemplifies the attention to detail required when dealing with hearing impaired children. The Glossary summarizes the various tests, for ready reference purposes.

## Types of hearing loss

How the different types of hearing losses already referred to are detected by tests is explained.

## Audiograms

Several audiograms are presented to illustrate common types of loss.

## Interpretation of audiograms

# The ear

## Why do we have ears?

In evolutionary terms hearing is more important than sight. Aquatic mammals have large parts of their brains devoted to the analysis of touch and sound. In oceans, with the absence of obvious boundaries, hearing is a social sense. The sounds made by individuals bind the group together. They are used to warn of dangers, to communicate feelings and to extend invitations. The same is true for humans. In our case speech serves the unique additional function of transmitting detailed knowledge from one generation to the next. Anything which affects hearing diminishes the individual's ability to learn language, speak, communicate and be a wholly untrammelled participant in the community.

Nature is said to be parsimonious. There is always some very practical and beneficial purpose for every structure in terms of function, with nothing being wasted or present in excess. The stapedius muscle has a higher ratio of nerves to muscle fibre than any other muscle in the body. This snippet of information is given by way of introduction. Without going into too much detail a general description of the ear and the way it works has to be given to convey some idea of the ear's complexity. The reader may then more readily appreciate why when it comes to educating the hearing impaired, because there has been a reduction in what nature considers to be a minimum to maintain average function, it is almost inevitable that there will be some deficit in terms of what is attained by hearing impaired children.

Among their number must be included some children with monaural hearing loss: such children may have a loss in one ear that is virtually total. It is generally said, even by specialists, that if hearing in one ear is normal, a loss in the other ear is unimportant. Over the years I have seen a number of children for whom it has been a disabling condition. Obviously the total amount of auditory experience is diminished. There are also certain occasions when important messages are not heard. A recent case illustrated this. The living room in the boy's home was arranged in such a way that he typically sat with his good ear nearer the television set. His mother complained about his not listening to her. The same sort of thing happened when they walked along the road. She held his hand on the deaf side, so his good ear picked up all the traffic noise. Such situations often arise during young children's parallel play, when one child talks about what he is doing, with the intention of being overheard. The reader will be able to think of many similar occasions. So, it is clear that children with monaural hearing have far fewer opportunities of hearing accurately and learning than children with two good ears. One further point is that the absence of correct functioning in *both* ears prevents the listener from paying attention to particular sounds of interest, when they are partly masked by background noise: the ability to do this is often essential (at a party, for example) and only possible because we can focus our listening. The muscles of the middle ear (see Figure 1) appear to allow our ears to 'lock onto' sounds coming from a particular point – in the same way as the muscles behind the eye move the eye to focus in the right direction.

In some quarters the so-called 'deficit model' (described above) is greeted with hoots of derision. As a counter it will simply be pointed out by way of example, that notwithstanding high standards attained by physically disabled people, the fact there is some deficit inevitably means an inability to compete on equal terms in sporting events with those who are at a pinnacle of overall fitness. This might seem so self-evident as not to be worthy of mention, but given the extraordinary fads that afflict the educational system from time to time, the current tendency to summarily dismiss deficit models and the information that can be gleaned from them, cannot be passed up without comment. Karl Popper pointed out decades ago that positive information can only be gained from negative instances. The implications embraced and productively acted on in most other disciplines are too seldom heeded in educational circles.

## The mechanics of the ear

Most people think of the ear as the rather convoluted piece that sticks out sideways from the head. This is generally known not to be the part that actually does the work, though in domestic pets it is obvious from the way they prick up their ears, the pinna, as it is called, helps with the detection of sound. Reference to the diagram of the ear (Figure 1) will explain the nature and effects of some types of hearing loss.

## Detection and analysis of sound

The way we detect and make sense of sounds is very sophisticated. Sounds produced by speaking, playing musical instruments, or everyday events radi-

Figure 1: Diagram of the ear

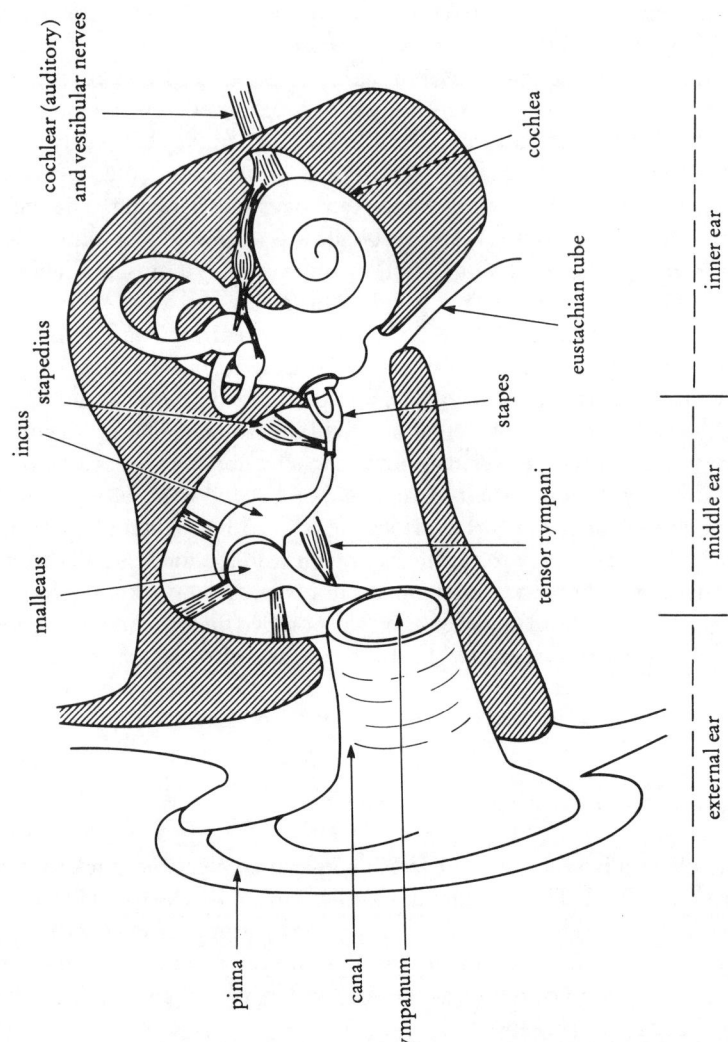

ate from the source. They are collected into the pinna. This leads into the auditory canal which terminates at the ear-drum (*tympanum*). As the sound waves strike the drum they make it vibrate. This vibration is transferred to the *ossicular chain* via the plate of the *malleus,* the first of the three *ossicles* (literally little bones). The movement of the malleus is transferred to the *incus* (anvil) and on to the *stapes* (stirrup – also named after its shape). The movements initiated by the vibration of the ear-drum reach the cochlear by means of the now oscillating disc at the end of the stapes, fitted against the oval window (*fenestra ovalis*). Pressure waves are induced in the fluid of the cochlear by the oscillations of the stapes. Up to this point the transmission of sound is mechanical in nature. The induced pressure waves in the fluid of the cochlear vary in length and are detected in different parts of the cochlear according to their pitch. At that point the physical movement is transformed into electrical nervous impulses. These travel up the auditory nerve to the *auditory projection areas* of the brain, that is the parts that make sense of what we hear.

This is by no means the whole story. As has already been pointed out the stapedius muscle is so positioned as to have very large effects on the way the ossicular chain vibrates. The tiny contractions by the stapedius muscle can distort the movements of the ossicular chain. In addition the *tensor tympani* is able to tighten the ear-drum, making it more sensitive to high frequency sounds. These two muscles interact in such a way as to preferentially tune the ear to detect speech sounds, especially the high frequency consonants that are so essential to the understanding of the spoken word. For these two little muscles to react in the way described there must be no hindrance to their movement. Everything must happen in milliseconds. First, some sound is detected and a primary analysis made. The brain has to send back messages to the muscles and they in turn modify the way in which the ossicular chain moves to aid analysis of subsequent sounds heard. This is why calling somebody's name to alert them has the effect of priming the auditory system to be ready for ensuing messages.

Apart from the bare bones described above, the entire auditory structure has all sorts of additional, inbuilt checks and balances to amplify very small sounds that may be of importance or to dampen down sounds which are so loud as to cause damage and overwhelm the entire system. There is also another activity of the ear that is seldom mentioned. Apart from *receiving* and analysing sound, the ear also *produces* sound. The brain sends signals to the stapedius and sensor tympani, which vibrate the drive and thereby make sounds. These can be detected by a small, sensitive microphone being inserted in the canal. *Oto-acoustic emissions,* as they are called, probably help with the analysis of sounds, speech in particular, due to the way in which they resonate with the incoming signals.

So it will be appreciated that the ear is not simply a passive receiver, it actively sends out signals. They are always absent when there is a conductive hearing loss (see below). In my experience children who have had this sort of hearing loss when young often have difficulty in learning a second language later. It may be that their ears are unable to send out the resonating signals which enhance the precise discrimination of unfamiliar sounds. It might also account for the quite disproportionately large effect of some seemingly mild losses. Staff in most Audiology Clinics have seen many children about whom parents, Speech Therapists and teachers have expressed concern. Yet after examination a report will have been given stating, 'Hearing within normal limits', often abbreviated to HWNL. It is virtually certain that nearly every class will have at least one child in this category – just a bit slow, not always trying hard enough. To date no specific research has been conducted on the relationship between oto-acoustic emissions, auditory discrimination and rates of learning. When it is, it is probable that the function of the two weak little muscles of the middle ear will be revealed as essential for quick accurate perception of speech and the learning that results therefrom.

## Hearing tests

The first type of tests used with very young children are called *distraction tests.* These are normally used up to about 18 months of age, or with the developmentally young. They depend on *reflex* responses. The child turns in the direction of the sound automatically. Typically the child will be seated on mother's lap. At first quiet sounds are made at a distance of three feet from either ear. The sounds may be made in a variety of mechanical ways, e.g. twisting a specially constructed rattle or quietly striking chime bars. Quiet voiced sounds such as 'ah' and 's' remain among some of the most reliable for testing the hearing of young children. *Pure tones* are also used when appropriate. These are made by a *free field audiometer.* A child with a very severe hearing loss may not hear any of these sounds and only respond to a drum being banged loudly. More details as to just how these tests are conducted may be found in the book by B. McCormick (1988).

When children are older they are given *performance (cooperative) tests,* so called because the child has to make a *voluntary* response when a sound (or word) is heard. In the case of a pure tone, inserting a peg into a board is an easy response. For a *speech discrimination test* such as the Kendal or McCormick Toy Tests, a miniature object must be pointed to when the name is spoken by the tester. With pure tones the results are recorded on an audiogram. In the case of the toy tests the loudness of the tester's voice is recorded. Just how loudly the tester is speaking is measured by means of a sound level meter, placed close to the child's ear.

The most accurate type form of performance test involves wearing headphones and is referred to as closed circuit. Some children as young as 18 months have sufficient confidence to accept a headset. The person testing judges whether or not to proffer the headphones to a very young child. As with the free field test, a voluntary response has to be made when a sound is heard. Older children and adults use a plunger switch which turns on a little light for the tester to see. This is more acceptable to mature individuals.

Another type of test, which does not call for any deliberate response from the subject is the *impedance bridge*. This is a quick and easy way of checking whether the ear drum is moving normally. A probe, with a soft plastic seal, is put against the canal and the air in it first sucked then blown, drawing the drum gently out or bulging it inwards. At the same time a sound is fed in. Changes in the sound are measured. This works on the same principle as a trombone or other wind instrument. The longer or shorter the length of tube, the lower or higher the sound. To conclude the test a louder sound is made to induce the stapedial reflex. A really loud sound elicits a reflex response in the stapedial muscle, a bit like a knee jerk. This is a very crude check of an abnormal response by the stapedius and provides no indication whatsoever of the finer functions mentioned earlier. With modern impedance bridges the results are printed out automatically (see Figure 2). The printout on the left shows normal compliance, i.e. the drum and the ossicles are all moving normally. On the right the line drawn is flat. This could be because: the ear-drum is stiff, as a result of the middle ear being full of fluid; all the air has been absorbed because the Eustachian tube is blocked or the ear-drum is perforated. Visual inspection, using an otoscope, would reveal which of these conditions is responsible.

Figure 2: Impedance printouts

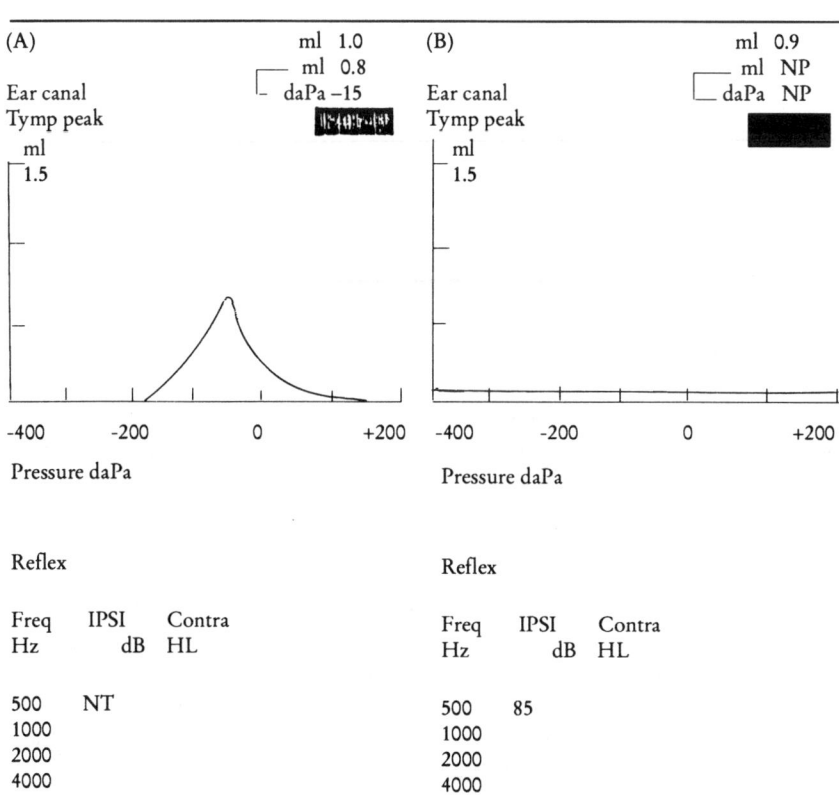

There are other conditions which would not be revealed in this way, but those described are the most common.

## Speech discrimination

When a full audiological assessment is conducted, speech discrimination will be investigated. This provides a check for the results of pure-tone audiometry, apart from being useful in its own right. How well a child understands speech is indicated by the accuracy with which words can be repeated. There are two sets of word lists commonly used. Their main characteristic is that each group contains words which contain the same vowel sounds but different consonants, namely brush/cup, tree/key, fish/ship. Typically the results will be given in the following format:

AB Word List

| | |
|---|---|
| Without aid (no lip reading) | 27% |
| Without aid + lip reading | 45% |
| With aid (no lip reading) | 60% |
| With aid + lip reading | 90% |

Very occasionally a Speech Discrimination curve will be plotted out, giving the results for different sound levels. The figures given above are not actual results though not atypical. Remember they will have been obtained in the ideal listening conditions of an audiology clinic. Such results cannot be obtained in the poorer acoustic conditions of most classrooms.

## Types of hearing loss

The most common cause of hearing loss in the young is conductive in origin. *Conductive* hearing loss is caused by anything which impedes the passage of sounds down the canal to the tympanum and mechanical transmission by the ossicles, across to the inner ear. In its most minor and transient form it can be caused by a build-up of wax which is easily syringed out. A heavy cold may block the *eustachian tube* connecting the back of the throat to the middle ear. When this happens the air in the middle ear is absorbed, pulling the ear-drum inwards and preventing proper movement and the normal function of the two little muscles. Imagine what it would be like if your eyeballs got stuck and instead of being able to swivel them you had to move your whole head to scan. Reading would be a very tiresome affair. Having the ear-drum jammed and unable to move freely is to hearing what the inability to move the eyeballs would be to seeing.

Most people are familiar with a change of altitude affecting the pressure in the middle ear. The act of swallowing normally corrects the situation, by either forcing more air up or allowing some to escape. Unfortunately conductive hearing losses caused by infections cannot be cured so simply because an infection interferes with the normal functioning of the ear. *Otitis media* may be the cause of the infection. This usually leads to a build-up of infected secretions which sooner or later burst through the ear-drum. When this happens the discharge can be seen running out of the ear and frequently has a nasty smell.

A common cause of mild hearing loss in childhood is a condition known as *'glue ear'*. A thick, sticky secretion builds up in the middle ear and prevents the normal mobility of the drum and ossicles. This and other types of secretion, caused by bacterial or viral infection, can be removed surgically. A small incision is made in the ear-drum. The glue can then be pulled out through the hole or infected secretions drained. The operation itself is referred to as *myringotomy*. After such operations grommets – little plastic spindles with a hole through the middle – are put through the ear-drum, to allow for drainage and keep the air pressure in the middle ear normal. After a time the grommets fall out as the skin of the ear-drum grows again, closing the hole. When a perforation is caused either surgically or by infection, some scarring of the ear-drum results. This reduces the sensitivity of the drum to varying degrees and can in some cases lead to a significant hearing loss. In some children who have chronic otitis media, which causes the ear-drum to be repeatedly perforated, the skin does not always heal and *tympanoplasty* (skin graft) might be carried out at teenage. One mother, who had misheard what the ENT Consultant had said, told the Appointments Secretary that her daughter had to come back later for a plastic ear.

A less common form of conductive hearing loss is caused by *oto-sclerosis*. This is like osteo-arthritis of the third little bone in the ossicular chain which causes the stapes to fuse with the surrounding bone of the oval window. It is normally more frequent in older people, though it may be encountered in children from time to time especially round about the time of puberty. Oto-sclerosis can be cured for a time by surgery but is almost certain to recur.

All types of conductive hearing loss that affect the normal movement of the ear-drum and ossicular chain prevent the two tiny muscles in the middle ear from doing their work properly and interfere with the correct, instantaneous analysis of sound. Medically speaking this is often considered to be 'not significant', but it can have quite severe, long-term educational implications, due to the child not hearing properly, a little bit here and a little bit there. All the little bits add up over years to a sizeable deficit.

Whereas most types of conductive loss can be treated, the same is not true of sensori-neural hearing loss, though some successful work is being done with cochlear implants. Cochlear implants involve surgery. An electrode is threaded into the cochlear. The electrode is attached to a receiver, embedded in the bone of the skull. The skin is sewn back over. An aid, much like an ordinary hearing aid is worn, but a magnetic emitter sits over the receiver and sends signals through the intervening layer of skin. At present cochlear implants are only of value to people who have lost their hearing and previously had normal speech and language development, to an adult level. Since a prolonged and intensive programme of learning is needed, following the implant, not everyone with an acquired, profound loss is a suitable case for treatment.

Sensori-neural hearing loss is caused by damage to the nerves in the inner ear or at some other part of the auditory pathway, possibly in the brain itself – so called *central deafness.* Some children who can detect sound normally cannot make any sense of what they hear. They are *aphasic.* Because they need such specialized educational provision it is very unlikely a truly aphasic child will ever be encountered in a normal school setting. Such children have normal acuity, that is, they can detect sounds as well as anyone else. It is the function, the ability to make sense of what is heard, that is impaired. As with hearing impairment there are varying degrees of severity, so that some mildly aphasic or disphasic children, sometimes labelled language delayed or language disordered, are found in ordinary schools.

This distinction between acuity (detection) and function (understanding) easily explained in relation to hearing, is important because it is often encountered at other times in the educational process. Ideally acuity and function should correspond, as for example when a new mathematical concept is explained to a child. The demonstration and explanation might be seen and heard, but it does not register. This is frequently attributed to a lack of central function in the child's brain, the child in question being regarded as not having the capacity to learn. Individual's abilities do indeed differ, but in such a situation it would be as well to reconsider whether the child has the relevant experiences to assimilate the particular concept to be learned.

Sometimes a hearing loss is made up of two components, part conductive and part sensori-neural. It is then referred to as a *mixed hearing loss.* Conductive hearing losses are never greater than 60 decibels. Sensori-neural losses can range from slight to virtually total loss. The clinician always checks carefully what type of hearing loss a child has because a combination of a conductive and a sensori-neural loss may make a child profoundly hearing impaired. When the conductive element is treatable, and the sensori-neural loss is not too great, the child may subsequently be able to make good use of a hearing aid and learn speech and language largely through hearing.

In order to give some idea of the sort of loudness measured and recorded on audiograms a range is shown below. It must be pointed out that the way in which loudness is measured is in accordance with a logarithmic scale so that the change in the force of the sound striking the ear-drum to register a difference of 5 decibels between 95 and 100 is thousands of times greater than between 0 and 5.

Loudness of sounds

| | | |
|---|---|---|
| 0 | dbs | quietest sound heard by a young adult |
| 30 | dbs | barely audible speech |
| 65 | dbs | normal conversation at 3 feet |
| 80 | dbs | shout or orchestra playing ff |
| 90 | dbs | damagingly loud |
| 100 | dbs | very loud disco (close to the threshold of pain) |
| 120 | dbs | jet plane at close quarters |

(dbs = decibels)

## Audiograms

The audiograms shown in the pages that follow are illustrative of results obtained by pure tone audiometry. They are mainly obtained under closed-circuit (wearing headphones) conditions.

Figure 3: Blank audiogram

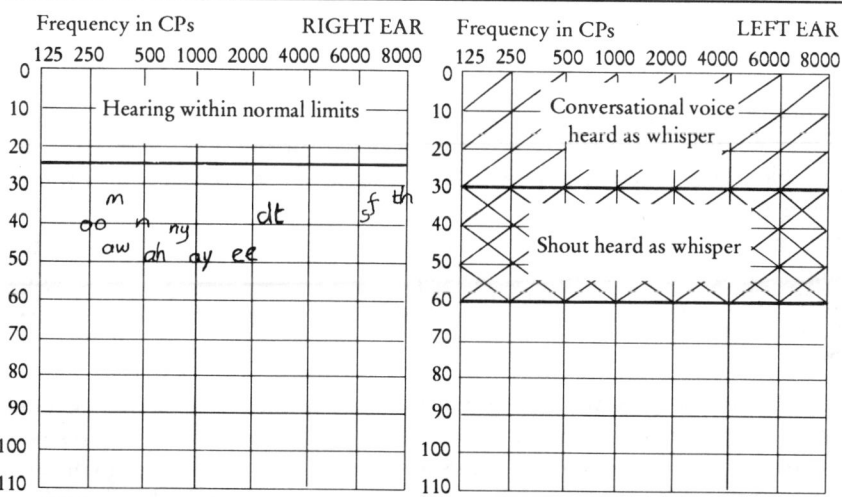

*Note:* The audiogram on the left shows losses up to 25 dbs, considered to be hearing within normal limits (HWNL). Also indicated are some speech sounds. Their position indicates their predominant frequency. The audiogram on the right shows that a loss of 30 dbs results in conversational speech being heard as a whisper. With a loss of 60 dbs a shout is just about heard.

Down the left hand side of the audiogram, loudness is indicated. At the top left hand corner is 0 decibels (dbs). This is the *threshold of detection*, i.e. the quietest sound a normal young person can hear. In the bottom left hand corner is 100 dbs. Because many audiograms span 0-100 dbs it has led some doctors to write reports in which they state the individual has a 40 per cent or maybe 50 per cent hearing loss. This is absolutely meaningless. It is now fairly rare to find such statements in reports but it is mentioned because it does still occur. A further piece of very misleading information sometimes included is the loudness of sounds heard when a very powerful hearing aid is being worn by the child. To the uninitiated it looks as though the child can hear almost normally, whereas all it really tells anybody is that the child can detect sounds amplified to such an extent that they would deafen a person with normal hearing. The blast of sound shakes the child's head so much that it knows a sound has been made from feeling and not hearing.

Across the top of the audiogram are the frequencies (cycles per second – cps) to be tested. 261.63 herz (that is close to 250 cps) is middle C on the piano. 125 cps is an octave lower. 500 cps is an octave above and so on for 1000 (1K), 2K, 4K and 8K. The range 250 cps to 1K encompasses the vowel sounds in speech. Above that are the consonants. It is in fact a lot more complicated than this, but this outline serves as an adequate guide. There is one additional feature, the line drawn all the way across at 25 dbs. Any response that is made between 0 dbs and 25 dbs is said 'to be within clinically normal limits'. This is a medical definition.

The frequencies routinely tested are: 250 cps; 500 cps; 1 K; 2 K; 4 K and 8K. 150 cps and 6K are usually omitted unless there is some particular reason for investigation. The procedure is to initially present a tone of 1K at a loudness previous observation of the child by the audiometrician has suggested will be heard. Then the loudness is reduced by 10 dbs. If a response is obtained the loudness is again reduced by 10 dbs. If a response is not obtained after reduction, volume is increased in 5 dbs steps (a change in loudness that is easily detectable). This lowering and increasing is repeated at each frequency for each ear in turn, to obtain the thresholds. It is a rather dreary procedure and maintaining the goodwill and cooperation of young children calls for skilful handling. As pointed out above careful, detailed observation, within a well-planned structure is essential both at the diagnostic stage and subsequently when teaching.

Before going on it must be pointed out that the ability to detect very quiet sounds is best at the time of birth. Then it is possible to hear bats squeak. Most people by the time they have reached their late teens can no longer do so. So the base line of 0 decibels represents a hearing loss for very young children, who can normally detect even quieter sounds of -10 dbs in the 4 K range (s, k, t, etc.). In normal speech the power of unvoiced consonants is much smaller than the power of consonants. They do not carry so well. We recognize that fact when attracting someone's attention at a distance. A loud, 'Oi !' does the trick. However hard you puff your cheeks, the same result cannot be obtained by using any of the unvoiced consonants. 'Psst' is a well-accepted way of attracting the attention of someone close at hand without alerting others.

Figure 4: Audiogram showing slight conductive loss

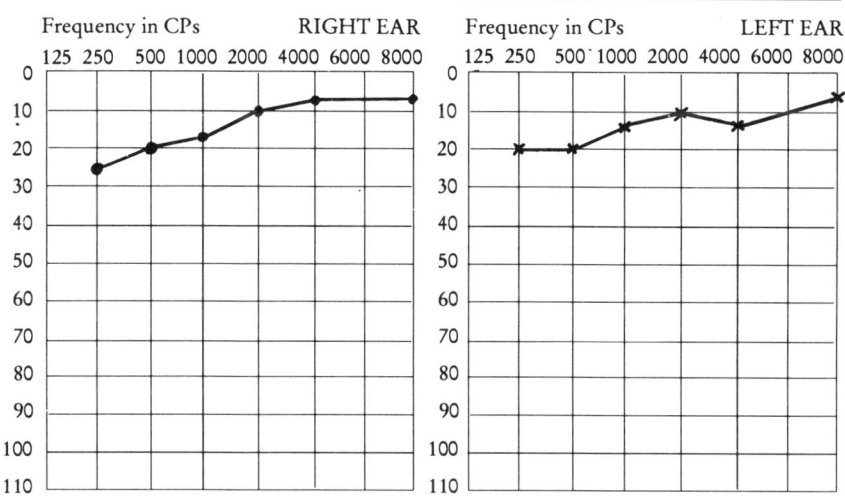

The sort of audiogram shown in Figure 4 might well be obtained in an audiology clinic or hospital, where hearing has been checked in good, quiet conditions, as a consequence of a child having failed a screening test in school or perhaps concern had been expressed about the child's ability to hear. This audiogram, because there is no loss greater than 25 dbs, is said to be within clinically normal limits. If an ENT (ear, nose and throat) surgeon looks and cannot see anything abnormal, the child will be discharged. Parents and teacher may well continue to be worried. The child does not behave as if everything is being heard all the time. As pointed out already young children have more sensitive hearing, especially for higher frequency sounds. Teachers and parents notice any diminished sensitivity in comparison with other children. As it does not constitute a 'medical problem' it is dismissed by doctors. In class there is the occasional failure to respond promptly. Information is often not remembered well, though sometimes, especially when teaching has been on an individual basis there is greater understanding and retention than when teaching has been in group situations. It is frustrating for the child and those with whom daily contact is made as 'something does not appear quite right.' In the face of expert opinion what else is there to be done? If the general principles given in Chapter 3 are followed there might well be a noticeable improvement.

On the audiogram shown in Figure 5, in addition to the circles, which indicate the *threshold of detection* for the right ear and the crosses for the left, there are also triangles. These are obtained by using a *bone conductor.* It is put on the mastoid process (the bony bump behind the ear) and the sounds produced by-pass the middle ear, stimulating the cochlear, via the bony skull. The position of the triangles show much quieter sounds were heard, on or close to 0 dbs. So there is a gap between what the child has the capacity to hear (i.e. the

Figure 5: Audiogram showing sensori-neutral hearing loss

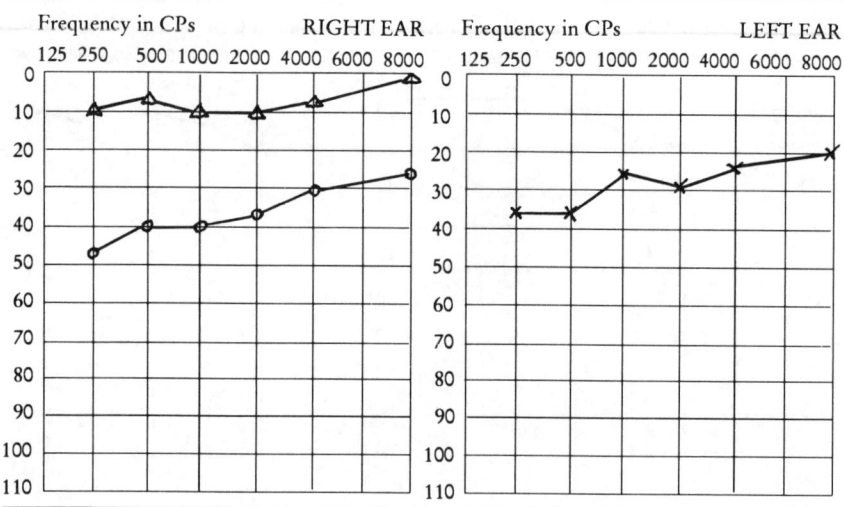

sensitivity of the nerves) and does hear. The audiogram reveals sound is not passing normally down the canal and across the middle ear. Possible reasons were given above. It may be wondered why no triangles were shown in the previous audiogram, said to illustrate a small conductive loss. Very often because the loss is no greater than 25 dbs, nobody bothers. With this mild/moderate loss it will often be evident that what is said is not heard properly. The child's own speech is likely to be free from any major defects, but ideas will not be expressed so easily and fluently as others of the same age. This characteristic frequently persists throughout school. One tedious way of checking the richness of a child's vocabulary and use of syntax is to record exactly what is said over a period of time and then break down the total into segments of 100 words. Each segment is analysed for how many new words are used. It is then found with children with limited vocabularies and restricted use of syntactical structures that with each successive segment the percentage of new words diminishes rapidly. So there may be 60 different words in the first, 20 new ones in the second and only a handful in the next and successive sections. Such methods are used primarily for research, but it is important to take note of the information it reveals with hearing impaired children if a suitable programme of instruction is to be devised.

The audiogram in Figure 6 shows that the individual has a lot of useful hearing, particularly for vowel sounds. There is a much greater loss in the higher frequencies, that is, for the consonants, especially the unvoiced ones (s, k, t, f, etc.). Such a loss is often described as a *ski-slope*, for obvious reasons. As the triangles are on or near the circles it shows the hearing loss is of sensori-neural origin, because there is no significant gap between air and bone conduction. There are further refinements and ways of indicating them on audiograms, but they are beyond the scope of this book.

Figure 6: Audiogram showing larger conductive loss

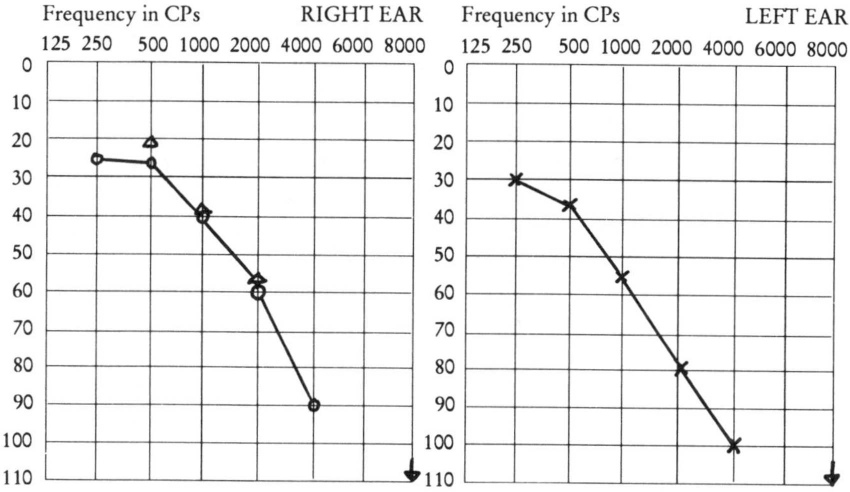

A child with a ski-slope loss often has defective speech. Vocabulary, knowledge and use of grammatical constructions are poorer than for the earlier forms and degrees of loss referred to. Individualized work schedules are of greater importance. Without carefully planned input more and more will not be heard, understood or learned.

## Interpreting the results

It is impossible to give an exhaustive interpretation of all the information which might be included in reports, but an outline of the main points will allow the most common features to be understood. It is assumed that the information was obtained in an audiology clinic, under good conditions, not simply 'Audio Test passed', which is the result obtained by a School Nurse doing routine *screening tests* in school.

It is unlikely that audiograms will be studied in great detail, together with all the implications for a child in an educational setting. What follows may be regarded as a rule of thumb so that the broad implications of what is recorded may be easily borne in mind and used for guidance.

## *All the responses on the audiogram are 10 dbs or better*

For whatever reason a hearing loss is suspected, any failure of the child to respond normally to sound is not due to any defect in the auditory mechanism. There are times when we all 'fail' to hear. We might be wrapped in our own thoughts or perhaps engrossed in a book. Fathers are less likely than mothers to hear a baby crying at night and respond. So occasional failure to take notice is normal. When it is more persistent or extreme, further investigations should be made.

I once saw a six-year-old child in a mainstream school, who appeared to be 'stone deaf'. He did not respond to anything said to him by anyone outside his field of vision. He was seen in an audiology clinic and issued with powerful hearing aids. These he refused to wear. Less powerful ones were substituted and these were tolerated. At that time I was working as a peripatetic teacher of the deaf. The boy's faultless articulation of the single words and short phrases convinced me he had either had normal hearing until very recently, or his hearing might possibly still be normal. The clue came by chance. I was taking him and his mother home after a visit to see the consultant who had issued the aids. At the bottom of the hill that led to their house the mother asked to be dropped off at the bottom. Her husband was of a very jealous disposition and always insisted he should be at home, even if only to let in the men who read the meters. Should a neighbour mention I had been seen dropping them off there would be all hell to pay.

Then I remembered an interview with both parents when the recent move to their present house had been mentioned. Formerly they had been in a small flat, with the boy sharing their bedroom. By some means it had been conveyed to him that what he could not see he must not hear. Working on this hypothesis I set up my teaching sessions in such a way as to persuade him he should respond, even when he was not in a position to 'lip read' what I was saying. Within a month the hearing aids had been discarded and his teacher had just one more 'normal' child in her class. That was perhaps the most dramatic and as it happened the most easily dealt with case of emotionally determined failure to hear. Most busy audiology clinics will have a handful of similar cases in the course of a year.

## Responses are on or between 25 dbs and 10 dbs

In the case of a mild conductive loss the sounds will probably have to be louder for low frequency sounds to be heard. A child with this sort of hearing loss could not and would not tolerate a hearing aid in a normal classroom. A normal conversational voice at a distance of three feet is about 65 dbs. Cutting off 25 dbs brings what is heard down to 40 dbs. This is like someone talking quietly – too quietly for comfortable listening. It is the sort of level that would lead an adult to switch off, unless what was being said was exceptionally interesting. There is, however, one further point to be remembered. As you move away from the child your voice gets softer. From one end of a big classroom to another this might be as much as another 20 dbs. Take those 20 dbs away too and the loudness of the sounds getting through to the child has been reduced to 15 dbs only. This is just loud enough to detect someone is talking, but not to understand.

'S/he hears when s/he wants to.' I wish I had a pound for every time I have heard that said about children with the sort of hearing loss being described.

The veracity of the statement has often been 'proved' to me. 'Jenny', the teacher calls loudly. Naturally a response is obtained (for the reasons explained above). 'Come here.' Jenny obeys. 'How old are you? When is your birthday? What's the colour of your dress?' These and other simple questions in similar vein are answered correctly. 'There you are! She can hear when she wants to. It's just that you're a bit lazy at times, aren't you Jenny?' I would like to be able to impose a £10 fine for that statement. Please remember the point that was stressed above about the muscles in the middle ear being prevented from functioning normally. If you saw a child with weak leg muscles, having difficulty with walking, you would think it cruel not to be considerate and helpful. Just because the muscles in the middle ear are small and invisible makes them no less important.

## Responses between 30 dbs and 55 dbs

It is possible that a loss of this magnitude could be caused by a conductive loss, but it is more likely to be sensori-neural or of a mixed type. If the child is not wearing a hearing aid, unless you are talking directly and providing the opportunities for lip reading, you might as well not be talking.

## Responses 55 dbs and more

In a normal classroom careful, specialized management of hearing aids is essential if the child is to hear what you are saying even when speaking, facing the child at a distance of three feet. Understanding of speech will virtually always have to be supplemented by lip reading.

## Responses in excess of 75 dbs at low frequencies only

Usually a teacher in a mainstream school will never encounter a child with a profound hearing loss of this severity, unless they are part of an experimental procedure; for local reasons there is no other provision or the parents have refused special education. There have been sporadic claims over the years for such children being taught successfully through hearing alone. The claims have usually been made in respect of girls at the age of three or four, when they have learned to say a limited number of words (hundreds) with reasonable clarity and been able to use short sentences. After that the publicity about their progress tends to die away, since it is usually not maintained (see Appendix A – historical perspectives for eighteenth century claims of a similar nature). It was mentioned earlier that the stapedial reflex occurs at about 80 dbs. This is caused by an abnormal spasm. The stapedius muscle's proper function is to delicately vary the tension of the ear-drum to help detect high frequency sounds better (s, k, t, f, etc.). A powerful hearing aid produces sound in excess of 80 dbs. The effect of sound at this level and above is to make the ossicles in the middle ear rotate, to protect the inner ear from damage. It is a purely mechanical re-action, due to the way in which the ear is constructed. It is therefore inevitable that any greatly amplified sound picked up by the inner ear is distorted. In any case since the higher frequencies are not being detected most consonants can-not be heard. Without these speech is unintelligible. Although hearing aids can help children with losses of this magnitude be aware of sound, they need con-sistent, full-time specialist teaching.

## The ski-slope hearing loss

What may be expected from children with this sort of loss varies considerably. It will depend to some extent where the drop-off starts. If the hearing loss is not more than about 40 dbs up to about 2K despite speech being mushy, lan-guage development may be quite good. Such an audiogram could look very similar to a slope that starts to drop away at 500 cps. But with the latter attain-ments are likely to be much poorer and instead of being mushy, speech might be almost unintelligible at times. The reason for the difference is that an ability to hear (amplified where necessary) up to 2K allows formants to be detected. Formants are those changes in sounds that we make as we slide from one phoneme to another. Formants give clues and make us ready to hear one type of speech sound more than another. Normally we are not aware of formants. Try saying slowly first, 'army', then 'ask'. You will find the 'ah' sound starts to break as you move your tongue into position for the 's' in 'ask'. This is ob-viously a very complex field and not something a mainstream classroom teacher can be expected to grapple with. The reason for mentioning it at all is because this type of loss can be so varied in its effect that what succeeds with one child fails completely with another. As a little twist in the tail, occasion-ally after dropping off dramatically in the middle frequencies, a child's hear-ing might be quite good at 8K. This improves speech discrimination markedly.

Children with ski-slope losses tend to provoke the most controversy about whether they can hear or whether they are shirking. Occasionally they will appear to hear everything that is said, especially if spoken to at close quarters. Some are very good at making the maximum use of information contained in formants and these are less easily detected at distances greater than a couple of feet. The murmur of conversation in an adjoining room gives some idea of how intelligibility drops off for such children.

## Potential symptoms of an undetected hearing loss

From time to time teachers suspect a hearing loss. It is seldom the symptoms accompanying enlarged tonsil and adenoids will be seen these days, i.e. the pinched expression, gaping mouth and difficulty with breathing. The symp-toms are likely to be of a less obvious kind. Instructions appear to be ignored or misheard. There is a restlessness whenever prolonged listening is called for.

Memory is poor. Occasionally a failure to respond is due to emotional reasons, as outlined above. One way of checking with younger children would be to play a little game in which they have to perform an action when a sound is heard. The response could be to stand, sit, touch their nose, etc., according to the instruction previously given. A xylophone gives a fair range and it can be struck very quietly. The teacher should take up a position behind the children, to avoid visual clues. It could then be seen if the child suspected of a hearing loss is consistently slower than the other children and getting the necessary clues from their movements. Another check could be made by calling a neighbouring child quietly, then seeing if the one you have doubts about responds to the same level, at the same distance (say 6–12 feet). Always remember the sounds used to check should be quite. Any checks should not appear unusual nor be repeated frequently, otherwise the child will start to feel different. Should the signs indicate a possible problem the school doctor can be asked to arrange further investigations. It is not unknown for information to already be on file but not passed on to the teacher.

# 3   Hearing Aids and their Management

The previous chapter gave some idea about the complexity of the ear, its function and the many variations in hearing loss that might be encountered. In this chapter the practical aspects of having a hearing impaired child in a mainstream class will be looked at in terms of hearing_aid management and how the teacher might need to behave differently when teaching hearing impaired children. First children with hearing losses who do not wear aids are considered.

A hearing impaired child may not wear an aid in an ordinary class setting for various reasons. The most likely one is because the loss is too small. When a slight hearing loss extends across the speech range, a hearing aid is unlikely to be of benefit in a normal classroom setting, due to *ambient noise*. Ambient noise is a combination of many different sounds arising from the activities within the room or outside. Some schools are in very noisy locations, perhaps near a busy road or close to flight paths of airports. Aeroplanes flying overhead can make conversation impossible at the best of times. The roar of the engines completely masks the sound of anyone speaking. For anyone, other than those with a profound loss, a hearing aid makes the row quite intolerable.

Even when a classroom appears to be reasonably quiet there is often background noise which is no longer noticed, but can easily be measured by a sound level meter. This sort of noise, habitually ignored by those with normal hearing, is picked up and amplified by a hearing aid making it more distracting. Consequently if a child with a mild hearing loss were to wear an aid the amplified ambient noise would be likely to mask speech to a greater or lesser extent. On one occasion I was trying to persuade a Headteacher of the effects of ambient noise on learning. She countered with her own experience of having gone to a school situated beside a noisy road. It had made no difference. She then recalled that she had not got such good grades as expected and only later gone on to get a good higher degree. There is always a danger in citing such anecdotal evidence, but over the years the pattern I have encountered has been remarkably consistent.

A second reason for an aid not being worn might be because a suitable aid cannot be fitted, for example for a child with a ski-slope type loss, hearing being near normal hearing up to about 2K in the speech range. There are certain to be some who will argue that it is perfectly possible to fit an appropriate aid for such a loss. In theory aids exist which can have low frequencies dampened down and high frequencies boosted. By selecting an appropriate elbow the high frequency output of the aid should be further enhanced. To ensure the least possible amount of precious high frequency amplification is frittered, the individual mould must have as short a projection as possible, with the maximum diameter hole in the middle. Unfortunately the theory does not match up to practice, despite manufacturers' claims. Identical models can vary greatly in terms of their performance. So unless a supplier is prepared to allow every aid in stock to be checked, there is no guarantee the specifications that come with the aid will be matched sufficiently for 'hard to fit' cases. If an aid is to be worn by such individuals, other than in suitably acoustically treated surrounding (that is carpeted, with sound absorbent materials on the walls and ceilings such as is found in special schools and Partially Hearing Units [PHUs]), it is likely the child will be very much less than keen to wear one. Ambient noise, especially the lower frequency components, makes amplification both uncomfortable and unhelpful. With the aid turned up enough to benefit from the amplification of the higher frequencies (s, k, f, t, etc.), extraneous noises are made unpleasantly loud. Even a jam-jar full of water for painting can startle if plonked down. There are usually in the course of the day many other such *impact noises*. At present, even though hearing aids can be modified to some extent, they all tend to amplify around 1K and that is the problem for children with the sort of loss referred to. In the majority of cases nothing can be done about either ambient noise or impact noises.

The third reason for not wearing an aid has already been mentioned. It is regarded as a stigma. This might be a personal response, not wanting to appear different, or due to parental attitudes. This calls for very sensitive handling. Usually the peripatetic teacher will try to deal with it. Occasionally an educational psychologist will become involved. Unless there are additional emotional and behavioural problems it is unlikely a psychiatrist would consider tackling such a refusal. Sometimes children, who are shy about being the only one in a school with an aid, accept and benefit if transferred to a partially hearing unit, where there are others in the same position. This is not invariably the case and I know of at least one instance where a child attends his neighbourhood school in which a partially hearing unit is based but refuses to become involved with it or wear an aid.

The feelings of hearing impaired children are more easily hurt than other children and teachers need to be sensitive to this, avoiding any comment that highlights the disability unduly. In the normal course of events a reproach addressed to one of the other members of the class, such as 'I don't think you were listening carefully', might well be justified and acceptable to the individual concerned. The same remark directed at a hearing impaired child could provoke an angry or tearful response. On the other hand, telling a hearing impaired child to listen carefully is quite appropriate, when it forms part of a normal and natural introductory instruction. In settings where all the children have a similar disability it is often possible to give instructions and make remarks that would be perceived as hurtful elsewhere. The community of experience facilitates a fairly direct approach, the intention being appreciated as aimed at a general improvement in the skills of all, not a criticism of one person in particular.

Children can be issued with many different kinds of aid. Companies that make aids produce a range to cater for various types and degree of hearing loss. Each company naturally claims better features than those made by others. The common characteristics of most of them are set out below.

# Types of hearing aid

## Individual aids

One or two hearing aids may be worn. In a mainstream setting the type is almost certain to be of the ear-level kind, though it might be used in conjunction with a radio-aid (see below). Each aid has three parts. The main body contains the works:

- receiver
- amplifier
- microphone
- battery
- on/off switch and 't' position

Nothing can be done with this part, other than changing the battery and checking the position of the switch. A plastic elbow screws onto the body. When the aid was issued the most appropriate sort will have been provided to ensure the best performance for the individual – as specified when talking about the 'hard to fit' child. So even though they may look the same to the layman they are not freely interchangeable. Attached to the elbow is a specially manufactured ear-mould, made to fit precisely. This should be checked daily to ensure it is clean and not blocked with wax. As young children grow these have to be replaced periodically. Badly fitting moulds make the aid squeal. This is not only annoying to others, it indicates that the child cannot be hearing anything of value, like incorrectly placed public address systems. The high-pitched squeal is caused by feedback from the microphone to the receiver. When it does occur the child should be asked to check that the mould is inserted fully. Very young children may need help to do this. We have all been told never to poke anything larger than your elbow into the ear (at least everybody connected with audiology), so most adults are hesitant about pushing in an ear mould. It is rather like being faced with a self-assembly kit. Firm, but gentle patience soon reveals the knack.

Individual, ear-level aids are small and light and can often be completely concealed by longer hair-styles. This does not affect performance. The most effective performance is obtained by the child being about three feet from whoever is talking to him or her. Ideally there should be a minimal amount of ambient noise and an absence of any large expanses of flat, hard surfaces which reflect sound. Such expanses, especially if coupled with a high ceiling, create a very reverberatory situation. Anyone wearing an aid in such conditions receives sound as if in an echo-chamber. Experiments have shown that even people with normal hearing cannot discriminate 100 per cent accurately if fitted with an aid in such conditions. This is the reason elderly people often only wear their aids in quiet domestic settings. Elsewhere the reverberations are such as to make listening more difficult. The sound is made louder, but more indistinct. It is unlikely that any individual teacher can radically alter the characteristic of the classroom, but any small area with soft furnishing and padded screens to the side will help to some extent.

## *Radio aid – Type 1*

Radio aids improve the quality of what the child hears markedly as soon as the distance from the teacher is more than three feet. The teacher has to wear a microphone. Due to its size and because it does not impede the teacher in any way, there is hardly ever any objection to the wearing of one, though it is not unknown for individual teachers to grumble and not use them as effectively as possible. The only time a teacher might have a gripe is if by chance more than one child in the class has a radio aid and they are of different types, when it would be necessary to wear more than one microphone. The microphone transmits on a radio frequency, direct to the child's hearing aid. The receiver is much bigger and bulkier than the ear-level aid. It may fit into a pocket, but it is much more likely to have some form of harness. The parts of the aid are much the same as the ear-level aid, but instead of the microphone (button) being incorporated in the body of the aid, it is on the end of a wire. The ear-mould clips onto the button. A further different feature is that the battery has to be charged daily. The advantage of radio aids is that the microphone is close to the speaker's, usually the teacher's mouth. Consequently ambient noise is less of a problem. It does mean, however, that the child cannot hear its own voice when speaking, unless the microphone on the receiver is turned on. Then ambient noise immediately becomes a problem again. A child with a hearing loss is very much in a 'no win' situation. In addition to this the transmitter is not at an optimal distance whenever there is a group or class discussion. It is possible to pass the transmitter round, but this is potentially a very disruptive operation.

In practice the teacher uses the transmitter microphone for individual or group work where the child is involved. In those circumstances, unless the child is speaking, the personal microphone is turned off (switch position 'T'). At other times the child has the aid switched to 'On' and the teacher's transmitter is switched off, so as not to distract with the remarks being made to other children – unless there is a specific reason for wanting the hearing impaired child to hear too. This might depend on the sort of lesson or activity going on at any given time. If the child is settled to do some creative writing then it would be inappropriate for him or her to be disturbed by unrelated comments. With painting or some other forms of activity where remarks of general interest are likely to be made, overhearing can be beneficial. The teacher should always remember to switch off when leaving the room. Gossip in the staff-room can transmit very well, especially if other children want a listen.

There is a variant of what has been described above. The child may have to wear an induction loop that fits round the neck, often tucked under clothing

– which does not affect performance. For best reception the child's aid should be correctly aligned to the loop, which entails being in a fairly upright position. Lolling or leaning over when writing impairs efficiency, leading to distortion of the signal received and loss of power. This could result in the teacher asking if the aid is switched on and working properly, since normal responses might not be obtained in such circumstances.

## Radio aid – Type 2

This is in many ways the same as Type 1. The difference is the child has an amplifier with extensions that attach to individual aids. This ensures sound of the same quality is heard consistently. No two aids produce exactly the same tone and there is a belief that variations can affect rate of learning.

With both types of radio aid the various parts should be checked daily:

- Are batteries charged?
- Is the aid working correctly in the 'On' and 'T' positions? A colleague will need to help check as there will be feedback if this is attempted with the aid close to the microphone.
- Are ear-moulds clean and fitting properly?

## Checking for faults

If the aid is not working properly, first check the battery. A stock of batteries to fit the individual aid should be kept handy. For radio aids a spare should be kept if possible. The next most likely cause for the aid not working is a break in the wire leads and finally the button(s). It is advisable to make testing of the aid(s) a daily routine. When a defect that cannot be dealt with on the spot arises it will be necessary to send the aid for servicing. Speed of repair can vary considerably, so the child will have to make do with an individual aid in the meantime.

## Important principles

When a child with a hearing loss cannot or will not wear a hearing aid, what else should be done? In such situations it is only possible to observe certain principles that will hold for all hearing impaired children including those with aids. Always make the fullest possible use of hearing. Regularly check aids are working. Even when they are, though the child may be enabled to hear loud, what is heard may very well not be clear. So additional forms of input, to supplement the defective hearing are called for. In the majority of cases this will be lip reading. Lip reading is something of a misnomer. It is not simply the movements of the lips which give relevant information. The position of the tongue and movements of the throat are also important. This will be readily apparent if a 'g' and a 't' sound are made. So being in a position to see the speaker clearly is paramount.

It is abnormal to keep at a fixed distance from the person being spoken to, but in the case of hearing impaired children unusual steps do have to be taken to maximise their opportunities for learning. Some constant features are of importance, whether an aid is worn or not.

## Lighting

It must always be ensured that lighting is adequate to illuminate your face well. Standing with one's back to a window should be avoided. The glare, especially on a bright day will make it difficult to see your face clearly and lead to eye-strain.

## Distance

About three feet, or closer if working on the opposite side of a table, is good. Nowadays children are often expected to sit on the floor when listening to their teacher reading a story. This is bad for a hearing impaired child. Whenever possible the child should be able to look straight ahead. It is difficult enough to look fixedly anyway, without getting a crick in the neck into the bargain. A further point to remember is that teachers tend to be fairly mobile. Movement is often restricted during story times, but at others this will be less so. Keep in mind whether any movements made will make lip reading difficult or interrupt it completely. A very able hearing impaired child, on the roll of a partially hearing unit was integrated for mathematics. He had some quite spectacular temper tantrums. They were caused on each and every occasion by the teacher turning away to write on the blackboard and continuing to talk. Fortunately the child in question passed the examination to go to the Mary Hare Grammar school for Deaf Children, where the teachers would never behave in this way.

## Speaking clearly

This would seem to go without saying. When working as a peripatetic teacher of the deaf I introduced a new member of the team to a number of parents of young children under school age, while showing her the ropes. Later one of the parents asked me if teachers like us had special training in speaking. She said that both of us, 'talked like cut glass'. The feature she had noticed was the crisp articulation of the high-frequency consonants. This results from precision of articulatory movements. It should not be exaggerated, but the slightly slower delivery, as when addressing a large group and the slightly more careful enunciation does make lip reading much easier.

## *Limiting duration of verbal exposition*

An eye-blink is enough to miss a vital word. Blinking is necessary to keep the surface of the eye moist. So obviously HI children blink. Explanations are usually structured in such a way that attention does not need to be paid to each and every word. None the less a very controlled watching must be maintained. This imposes a strain. The occasional pause, as well as shorter duration over-all should be the aim. The writing of keywords can make natural breaks and allow relaxation. Either a blackboard or an overhead projector can be used. An advantage of the latter is there is no need to turn away from the class and the jotting down of words does not interrupt the flow unduly.

So much for what can be done in practical terms. The other aspects of teaching style that have to be modified are related to language. Since this is a field fraught with complexities and trapped like a minefield it is dealt with separately in the next chapter.

# 4 Speech and Language – General Issues

## General issues

Speech and language serve to free us from direct experience. They are the means by which knowledge is passed on from generation to generation. An equally important direct function is the teaching skills. This applies as much to practical techniques in infancy as to great refinement in art or musical endeavour later. They may also be used to convey to others abstract messages over and above what is contained in the individual words themselves. How the words are spoken and in what context can convert a positive statement into the opposite. Such supralinguistic characteristics of speech serve a large role in social development. To obtain a more comprehensive grasp of all that is entailed in these brief statements the reader needs to go to either basic texts on speech, language, syntax and thinking, or more advanced ones, depending on present level of knowledge.

When thinking of language it should not be forgotten that specific vocabulary and language structures help us to organise our thoughts. In science and mathematics many of the concepts entailed could not be communicated to others without closely defined, specialized terminology and symbols. As is stated in the proposals for the national curriculum, August 1988, 'Mathematics is the most abstract of subjects' (p. 14; 4.15). Two other quotations from the same document serve to indicate why mathematics cannot be considered separately from language skills.

> The Interim Report specified a sixth area of mathematics. This includes the mathematics of decision making, critical path analysis, logical relationships, network analysis, numerical methods, the development of algorithms and computer programming (p. 3; 2.7).

This is of course only information for teachers, children, at least at primary level are only expected to, 'Understand and use terms such as prime, square route, cube, multiples and factors' (p. 25).

An example given at this level is: 'Understands the programme:

```
10 FOR NUMBER = 1 TO 10
20 PRINT NUMBER*NUMBER
30 NEXT NUMBER'.
```

The reader needs to look at the proposals or the national curriculum itself as it becomes available to appreciate why no separate section dealing with mathematics has been included, since as the proposals state:

> We recommend that the National Curriculum Council give early attention to the development of course materials and teaching approaches designed, within the National Curriculum framework, to

help teachers to get the most out of the one sixth of their pupils with special educational needs (p. 89; 10.32).

All that can really be said about mathematics is that straightforward computational skills can be taught as easily to hearing impaired children as any others, provided the appropriate stages are followed. Modern mathematics, with its heavy dependency on language skills is a very different matter. Problem solving or any other mathematical skill that has to be explained by means of an unfamiliar vocabulary is not understood well, if at all by hearing impaired children. This is not an area on which guidance can be given. It is one that presents difficulties even to the specialist, a fact reflected in the dearth of references in the library of the Royal National Institute of the Deaf. Such little as there is is primarily concerned with what is done at the nursery and infant stages and that basically refers to good practice anyway. It is not proposed to detail this here as once again 'what' and to some extent 'how' will be set out in the national curriculum when it is issued in its final form. What follows is in the nature of a summary of the other extensive language fields referred to at the beginning.

It is first necessary to describe normal development so that the interfering effects of hearing impairment can be set against it. There is an unavoidable concentration on early stages, since the speech and language development of hearing impaired children is often significantly delayed. Without full cognizance of such delays, erroneous assumptions may be made, resulting in insufficient investigation into what is or is not known by a hearing impaired child. That is the scope of the first part of this chapter. The second half of the chapter is concerned with some of the ways a teacher can structure teaching approaches and styles to provide the best possible opportunities for a hearing impaired child to learn.

It will become clear from the first part that there may well be some insuperable problems either in a main stream or a special school setting. A word of caution: always be wary of any assertions that are made claiming a technique is the ultimate answer. I have attended many worthwhile lectures and conferences where very careful presentations have been made, the speakers detailing the contributions particular methods make to an overall approach. At others extravagant claims were made for particular methods. Some of these are no more than a tinkering round the edges. Hearing impairment exerts a profoundly pervasive effect on the development of language, which is such a vast and complex dynamic, that it is inevitable some features cannot be taught if the fundamental prerequisite – normal hearing – is absent.

The word 'language' is derived from the Latin word meaning tongue, since language in its primary form is spoken. Language has many varied forms, but its function is always the same; to convey information. What is not conveyed by the word is the underlying process. In the case of spoken language, the speaker has to structure thoughts and ideas, then convert them into a string of sounds. These sounds are heard by the listener who hopefully decodes them to have the same meaning as the speaker intended. This does not always happen, as when somebody exclaims, 'We are obviously talking at cross purposes'. The event if not the reaction is much more likely to happen when talking to a hearing impaired child.

Language is so much a part of our everyday lives and acquired so easily by most people that precisely what is involved in learning it, together with the necessary conditions entailed are seldom considered by anyone, other than specialists. As has already been mentioned and is abundantly clear to anyone who has had dealing with hearing impaired individuals, language acquisition constitutes an enormous hurdle for them.

It should not be thought that simply learning words and constructing sentences are the only problems confronting hearing impaired children. Learning language is inextricably intertwined with the processes of thinking and understanding. What is more, many hearing impaired children have difficulty in coping with what may be termed the uncertainty principle. They tend to store information in a much more discrete and compartmentalized fashion than their normally hearing peers. There is one among many psychological theories about how information is stored, in which the memory store is thought of as a whole series of cubby-holes. It certainly seems to fit the hearing impaired. As a result they tend to interpret everything in absolute terms. In practice this means refusing to accept any modification of anything taught earlier, in the event of its being recalled. This can prove a stumbling block, since information is often simplified when a subject is first introduced. It is modified later, once basic concepts have been assimilated.

The problems referred to may be illustrated by two types of examples. The first relates to social behaviour. Early in life children are often told to ask if they want something. In school the same may apply in respect of sharpening pencils, getting items of equipment, etc. Then comes the day when it is said that there is no need to ask, though there may still be an embargo on perhaps paint and certain types of paper. Most children have no difficulty in accepting the way in which the rules have been changed to take account of increased maturity and the need for personal responsibility. The hearing impaired child might well interpret the statement, 'There is no need to ask' as blanket permission, or what is more likely persist with former patterns of behaviour, irritating the adult in the process. Another example of this type relates to the generally accepted principle that if someone drops something or makes a mess in some way, the individual concerned deals with the situation. A hearing impaired child's reaction if asked to tidy up after someone else is often, 'I didn't do it'. It was in the context of making a mess that I vividly recall a girl dropping a quart (approximately 1 litre) bottle of ink. She looked down in horror at the broken glass, the spreading pool of ink and the splashes on herself and everything else in the vicinity, then up at me. 'Aren't you going to shout and get angry?' she gasped. It seemed inconceivable that I would not and the explanation that it had been an accident did not prevent her from continuing to steal glances, after the mess had been cleared up, to see whether the anticipated anger might not have surfaced after all.

Hearing impaired children have great difficulties in coming to grips with more abstract concepts. In Science, for example, the atom is said to be the smallest particle (of an element). Subsequent mention of smaller particles might either elicit annoyance that the truth was not told in the first place, or a rejection of the new information. Something of the kind occurred when I was teaching in a school. A boy had looked at a simple science book and told his teacher what he had read. His teacher said the boy had got a fact wrong. The boy's retort had been that he would come and ask me. I was bound to know (what he had said was right) because I was younger. At the most abstract level many social issues are encountered. It is wrong to kill. Yet in Social Studies arguments may be put forward about situations in which it is regarded as permissible. Hearing impaired children are likely to give up even trying to understanding such things and look bored or vacant. The teacher will soon be able to detect when attention has been switched off and take appropriate action – if possible.

# Language

In some quarters language is traditionally regarded as developing through three stages. The first which normally lasts from 0–9 months comprises the auditory and language experience stage. During this time there is absorption of information. Over the next nine months there is the emergence of single words. The end of the second stage is marked by the use of simple sentences. This leads into the third stage, in which increasing use is made of syntax, complex sentences and the whole range of the grammar of a mother tongue – some researchers maintain complete mastery is achieved just over the age of four.

## *Stage 1 – Auditory and language experience (0–9 months)*

The foundations for the learning of speech and language start to be laid before we are born. Sounds are heard in the womb. In the later stages of gestation they make the foetus move. The varied intonational patterns of the mother's voice are audible before birth. These are automatically analysed and discrimination of speech sounds (phonemes) starts. After birth the whole range of speech sounds are heard. Within days, high frequency speech sounds not heard in the womb are discriminated. The baby makes sounds itself. By a process of interaction between the proprioceptive feedback arising from its own vocalizations and what is heard, words are learned and eventually the whole spectrum of communication through speech. At this stage there is an immense amount of spontaneous vocalizations, together with the associated feedback and incidental exercise of the articulatory mechanisms, leading to ever greater mastery. Just how many hours any individual spends in babbling is not known. Furthermore the spontaneous vocalizations lead to adults interacting more, by way of response. Hearing impaired children tend to make less sounds and later say less and ask fewer questions. The implications of this are that once they reach school they have had very many fewer experiences and less of the practice needed to develop language normally. It is this deficit which forms the background for any teaching programme.

Congenital hearing losses or any losses acquired early in life have a more marked effect on speech and language development than those acquired later. Prematurity is likely to deprive the child of some pre-birth experiences, since the auditory mechanism has not been functioning for so long – or at all in the case of very premature babies. Furthermore, adverse conditions arise if the baby is placed in an incubator, where quite meaningless sounds will be heard in terms of speech and language development. Quite a lot of children with some degree of hearing loss and/or subsequent speech and language delay are premature babies.

Within days of birth it is evident babies are interested in their environment. Their attention is caught by novelties, especially as far as what they can see and hear is concerned. Very early on the interactive nature of seeing and hearing is apparent. Anything heard is looked for. Anything seen and grasped is explored for sound making possibilities. This lays the foundations for later behaviour. Hearing impaired children are less likely to explore the sound making potential of what they see. By failing to do so they do not pay such prolonged attention and may well overlook additional visual features continued exploration would reveal. The cumulative effect is a more limited experience of the visual world. Hearing impairment has a continuously depleting effect. So just how the development of other skills is affected by a hearing loss needs to be taken into account.

The activity, interest and willingness to learn displayed by babies is typical of any healthy individual. The same holds for wanting to learn more about what is already known. The extraordinary lengths some people are prepared to go in pursuit of hobbies and pastimes convinces one of this. Many adults who work with children in a professional capacity may well observe that they know children, adults too for that matter, for whom this does not apply. In practice, 'I'm not interested,' often means, 'I've tried before and learned from experience that I can't.' In such circumstances the way those who would be teachers (parents in this context) failed to structure the environment in a suitable way for learning to occur needs to be examined. Hearing impaired children are naturally at a disadvantage from an early stage because what are appropriate structures and approaches in normal circumstances are not so for them. In my experience some of the lack of motivation ascribed to hearing impaired children certainly stems from very early failure and frustration.

As adults we are usually unaware of the way our bodies resonate when we speak, especially the thorax and head, though the resonance can easily be detected by placing the palm of the hand just below the collar-bone and saying, 'Ah' or against the cheek when saying, 'm'. Early in life there is a much closer association between what is heard and felt. For this reason a baby can be made to coo and gurgle by gently rubbing its stomach, as readily as by cooing in return. The close link between sound and touch has been mentioned before and will be dealt with again later when the teaching of writing is treated. The various senses serve to reinforce each other. When one is absent others are weakened not strengthened, since part of the mutual support is lacking. It is a fallacy that the lack of one sense leads to the enhancement of another or that those who are not good with their brains are good with their hands. The way all the senses feed into understanding is shown in diagrammatic form.

Figure 7: Flow-chart showing reciprocal reactions involved in sensory perception and communication

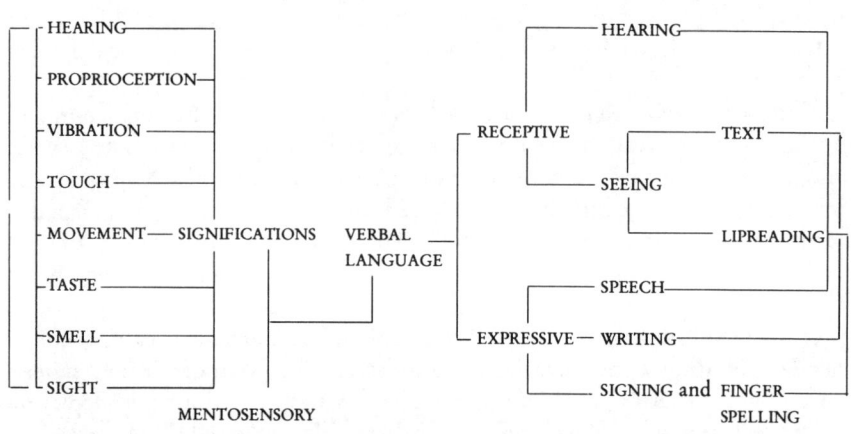

It will be noted that hearing and sight are shown as being antagonistic. Much of the time information from both can be integrated, but it is possible to be totally engrossed by one, to the exclusion of the other. This is a function of the central nervous system and not something that can be tampered with. One can never be aware of all the senses simultaneously, one sense always predominates. With some kinds of hearing loss children seem unable to achieve a normal balance. Their audiograms indicate what appears to be a lot of useful hearing. Yet speech and language is poor compared with children who have greater degrees of hearing loss. It might be that neither lip reading nor hearing is sufficiently good to follow what is said and so they fall between two stools, constantly switching from one sense to the other and gleaning insufficient from either to learn.

In the early stages of life a great deal of exploration goes on. The mouth is the primary organ. Everything goes into a baby's mouth. Later it is the exploring index finger that gets poked into anything pokeable. A wide variety of sensations are experienced: taste, smell, touch, movement. Usually a small range of objects are identified, almost equally by the senses just listed. The feeding of information into the brain from the senses is associated automatically. In this way significations are formed. Any familiar object may be described in terms of one or all of the senses. At some stage the familiar sensations relating to objects and events become associated with particular words being spoken.

The pattern of the sounds contained in the words is incorporated in the relevant signification and then it has the power to generate meaning in terms of personal experience. Later, when the word is heard in other contexts, it can elicit searching or anticipatory responses. Most people will have witnessed a baby pay attention when it hears a familiar word used by adults in an otherwise uninteresting conversation. It is also the reason some dog-owners spell out the word walk, as most dogs can't spell.

## *Stage 2 – Single words*

Usually the will precedes the skill. Emerging skills arise from maturational changes. When this does not happen, because one or more modalities are impaired, the individual (child) experiences a great deal of frustration. This is likely to arise early in life, when the ability to communicate normally fails to develop. Parents and other caretakers are also frustrated. We are programmed to expect certain skills to be acquired in an age related way. 'Don't be a baby', 'Act your age', etc., are everyday expressions of such attitudes. If in spite of persistent efforts success is not attained it is natural to give up.

The failing behind that may have started before birth continues as deprivation of the full range of normal auditory experiences continues. It happens for the following reasons. A baby spontaneously makes sounds. The nature of these sounds and the order in which they emerge are genetically determined. By and large open vowel sounds and sounds involving the lips (m/b/p) come first. These are followed by others where contact is made between the tongue and dental ridge (n/d/t/l/j), later speech sounds at the back of the throat (g/k) and finally sibilants (sh/s/z). Hearing impaired children, including those with profound losses, normally make most of these sounds. But if they are not heard clearly, either when made by the baby or by others, they are not repeated and practised. This has grave implications for the quality of their own speech later in life.

Before saying the first identifiable word, babies with normal hearing get a lot of articulatory practice. They derive pleasure from incorporating newly mastered sounds. The physical aspects of the activity exercises the lungs and leads to improved breath control. Many hearing impaired children have difficulty in controlling a stream of air. Those with a high frequency loss, apart from not hearing the sounds properly anyway, do not have the required degree of fine control of the diaphragm needed to produce crisp sibilants. Other speech sounds containing high frequencies are likely to be distorted or absent. Since these are the most important ones in English for intelligibility, it will be appreciated that a great swathe is cut through the words that can be understood and spoken.

As a rough guide any polysyllabic words that contain j, k, s and z, especially in combination, will be harder for hearing impaired children to hear, understand, learn and use themselves. The examples 'mustn't' and 'shouldn't' clearly fall into this category. Not only are they hard to hear, there is very little to see, from a lip reading point of view. A quick glance in a mirror when saying them will reveal how 'stn't' or 'dn't' elided in an indistinguishable way. It is not that these words should be avoided in school, only that *special care* is taken to ensure clear reception and understanding. Often the only way to clarify such words will be to actually write them.

The initial learning of individual words has the effect of crystallizing what has, up to then, been a rather formless amalgam of primary sensations (shown on the left of Figure 6). Words provide tags which facilitate recognition and retrieval of information from the memory store. As an integral part of significations words also have another function: they provide a framework that more readily facilitates the assimilation of new information. As vocabulary and language skills in general increase, a vast, exceedingly complex, enmeshed network evolves – making possible a wide variety of associations and thereby enabling the transfer of operations from one situation to another. Most readers will be familiar with these concepts from the work of Piaget. A good summary of the sensory-motor period development, as well as the stage of formal operations and perception, are contained in J.H. Flavell's book (Flavell, 1963); this is recommended reading to flesh out my necessarily brief description. Hearing impaired children miss out on part (or all) of the processes described in detail by Piaget; consequently, the firm links which are normally established between direct experiences and early language are weak or absent.

The way we use the sort of language network referred to above in order to retrieve and restructure what we know, can easily be illustrated by thinking in turn of: all fruits; tropical fruits; citrus fruits; imported fruits. These labels are sufficient to retrieve groups and subgroups, make comparisons and draw distinctions. A central feature of hearing impaired children's thinking is the slowness and difficulty that they have in doing this. Their capacity for analogic thought is almost always less than that of other children of the same age. For this reason do not assume explanations relying on this kind of thinking will be readily followed by them. An example of a failure to do so occurred when I was teaching young hearing impaired adults who wanted to improve their language skills. A short story had been chosen in which a reporter tried to gain an interview with an actress in a restaurant by asking her the time. She told him and repeated it when he attempted to pose other questions. Not one of those in the class caught on to the fact the reporter had been given the brush-off. This showed their failure to abstract the message not explicitly contained in the words.

Messages are also conveyed by supralinguistic features, i.e. not in either the words or the way in which they are used. Early on in life information is gained from tone of voice, the cooing of pleasure and the rasp of exasperation. Later much more subtle information is conveyed by the sarcastic comment or excited response. A quiet word could convey a serious warning, while loudness may simply signify pay attention. Naturally we modify our behaviour in response to how we are spoken to. If a list were made of variations in tone it would be very long: admonitory, disapproving, warning, and many more for each letter of the alphabet. The emotive content of a message can often be picked up without understanding the words spoken. The tone is often important when a child becomes independently mobile. But it is precisely then that the effects of even quite small hearing losses can start to have an ever greater impact. Increased distances are put between the child and whoever is speaking making it more probable that what is said will not be heard correctly or at all.

The responses made to different tones might be learned unconsciously, or perhaps be innate. Whatever the truth of the matter one thing is certain. To detect the subtleties and differentiate between the varying information contained in the tone as opposed to the content, hearing must be good. Even quite slight losses will affect accuracy in deciphering the hidden message, making unsafe assumptions that additional information will be conveyed by changing the inflection of the voice. With most children talking quietly, using a cold tone indicates anger and annoyance, possibly a warning. A child with a hearing aid is simply likely to turn it up a little to hear you better. So it will be appreciated how certain socialization functions of supralinguistic features may fail to be effective.

## Stage 3 – Simple sentences and the emergence of more complex features

The reason for all the emphasis on very early development has already been given. What has not been made clear is the way hearing impairment insidiously and exponentially exerts its affect on speech and language development. It can lead to a delay of months or even years compared with normal development. Therefore it cannot be taken for granted that by the time a hearing impaired child starts at school all of the most basic vocabulary and language structures have been learned. The most that can be expected is that he or she has sufficient receptive and expressive language skills to cope in a mainstream setting – though this is by no means certain. A knowledge of the general pattern of language development will serve to make any gaps more apparent. To begin with certain core features are presented in Table 1 (see page 48).

A cursory examination of Table 1 is sufficient to reveal how the earliest concepts and vocabulary relate to self. Prior to recognition of one's own name there has been extensive exploration of the body. Varied activities such as the sucking of fingers, playing with toes, poking fingers into any intriguing orifice, have led to an awareness of what is self and not self. There is also the recognition of relationships between the self, objects and people. Once individuality is established dyadic relationships (we, us) are understood. As decentering continues pronouns which indicate relationships between others (you, them, theirs) make sense. The earliest inkling of fairness emerges around the same time. What applies to self is understood to apply to others and vice versa. Depending of the severity of the loss hearing impaired children may lag months or years behind in the learning of these concepts.

**Table 1: Vocabulary learned by most children in the first five years of life**

| Age (years) | | Knows | |
|---|---|---|---|
| 1 | own name | | |
| 1$^1$/2 | mummy, daddy, names of sibs | me, mine, my, this, | |
| 2 | nan, brother, sister | mummy's, daddy's, etc. | |
| 2$^1$/2 | uncle, aunt | I, you, ours, that, it, | |
| 3 | friend | we, he, she, they, yours, | |
| 3$^1$/2 | cousin, family | her, him, them, | |
| 4 | | his, hers, theirs, | age and names of teacher and classmates |
| 4$^1$/2 | | | names of other teachers |
| 5 | | | address, birthday |

Some of the facts listed later are not different in kind from the earliest ones, for example, the names of other teachers and home address. Date of birth is much more abstract, encompassing a very long time-scale for a young child. As has been repeated time and again, hearing impaired children often have much more difficulty in learning and understanding anything which has abstract features. For this reason it is important to actually check personal pronouns are known and understood. Similarly attention should be drawn to various features of the calendar. This needs to be done on a daily basis. By making references to, actually displaying where necessary, work which has been done before, helps to establish the dimension of time, as well as reinforcing by recall what has been previously learned. Retrieval of information – because it is unlikely to have been so securely learned in the first place – is always more difficult for hearing impaired children. Therefore any ploy to establish continuity and make knowledge more readily accessible for recall should be used.

Due to the variable and unpredictable way in which hearing impaired children miss out on language experiences their language development tends to be patchy. A similar situation can be encountered in children who have had very little verbal stimulation. As far as the latter are concerned, provided their hearing is normal, once they are in a more stimulating setting many of these gaps are filled in spontaneously, making a detailed analysis unnecessary. Such an analysis is, however, necessary with hearing impaired children. Once more a table that starts at the lowest level is included to illustrate the beginning with words of personal relevance spreading out to include words given by way of instruction, once the child is acting independently, especially within a group (Table 2).

48

**Table 2: Common nouns, verbs, adverbs, adjectives, prepositions, wh- questions**

| Age (years) | Nouns | Understands Verbs | Adverbs/adjectives | Prepositions/ questions |
|---|---|---|---|---|
| 1 | mouth, eyes, cup, spoon, drink | stand, stop, cry, look, take, | more, naughty, | up, down, whose |
| $1^1/2$ | hands, feet, chair, table, door, | give, eat, 'wanna' | good, | on, what, |
| 2 | nose, ears, hair, finger, (*common objects:* flower, car, telephone, knife, etc.) | blow, brush, close, -n't, watch, hide, find, sleep, show, | common, colours | in, beside, where |
| $2^1/2$ | teeth, knee, tongue, fork, toes, (*items of clothing:* sock, coat, hat, etc.) | bite, listen, taste | nice | by, which |
| 3 | tummy, bottom, head, flag, (*names of animals:* cat, dog, horse, etc.) | put, make, look, -ing, scratch, fly, run, | big, nasty, brave, little | under |
| $3^1/2$ | elbow, palm, waist, shoulder, thumb, leg, numbers 1–10 | hold, step, jump, hurry, | quick, slow, quiet | behind, when, together |
| 4 | days of week | cook, carry, shine, buy | tight, careful, | near, how, why |
| $4^1/2$ | house, window, chimney | | gentle, right, wrong | apart |
| 5 | (can define words) | | same, different | |

*Note:* Usually children can use words and grammatical construction 6–9 months after they are understood.

Children vary considerably as to the exact vocabulary they acquire and the order in which they do so. The examples given above are some of those most commonly learned. In the table types of immature contractions and contractions of the negative are included. Although the adult form may be: 'want it' the child will at first say, 'wanna' and 'gonna' instead of 'going to'. Also the contracted forms 'can't', 'won't' and 'isn't' emerge first. At a transitional stage a child will often expand a contracted negative to be more emphatic. The following example was recorded when a child (with normal hearing) was about to be forced to do something he did not want.

(1) 'I don' wanna', (2) 'I don' want to', (3) 'I don't want to'.

This illustrates the use of both tone and attention to precision of articulation to convey feelings. They add another dimension to the basic message. Notice how the sounds initially omitted are the high frequency, unvoiced consonants, precisely the sounds many hearing impaired children cannot hear well or at all in some cases.

As would be expected nouns predominate over other kinds of words. Even in this area hearing impaired children will have a much more limited range. Some idea of the effect of hearing loss on the acquisition of passive vocabulary may be gained from the fact that in their mid-teens many profoundly hearing impaired children know about as many nouns as a $3^1/2$ year-old child with normal hearing. Those with a moderate/severe loss often do not get beyond about an 8 year-old level. Excluded from this generalization are words which might have been taught quite specifically in relation to specialized subjects, especially at secondary level. Even when words are understood they may not be used when speaking and writing. Consequently a lack of fluency of expression is commonplace.

It will be noted that an ability to define words is included at a 5 year-old level. Often the definitions given at this age are in simple terms, e.g. a hat – goes on the head; a nuisance – gets on your nerves. Many hearing impaired children do not get beyond this stage, because to give more detailed and general definitions calls for a large vocabulary. Due to their limited vocabulary, if called upon to do any creative writing, many tend to be very repetitive. Often the same vocabulary and simple narrative constructions will be used over and over again. Unless all the work produced is periodically reviewed as a continuum, individual pieces may look acceptable, but considered as a whole there has been very little progress over time. Language enrichment has to be quite deliberately and consciously planned, since all the incidental learning which is the norm does not happen to the same extent.

Now some more examples of the early mastery of language by young children is given in Table 3. Compare the examples quoted with the two following verbal descriptions of pictures by profoundly hearing impaired children,

> 'The man eat knife. The man look at the man because the man was sitting on the chair with the table.' (15 year-old girl)

> 'The man sleep the bed. Mum said, 'Come eat breakfast.' He said, 'No, thank you.' Tired. Sleeping. Weather shining.' (14 year-old boy)

Two further examples illustrate conversational abilities.

> 'We are going to museum with Mr. X. Then we have a look at the picture. Then we go back to dining room. Finished.' (Account of the day's events, 13 year-old boy)

> 'About a boy went chocolate factory. Then the boy big peach.' (14 year-old girl's attempt to recount a book she had read)

Table 3: Language structures

---

**1 year – single words**
This is mainly naming, though it can indicate a want, e.g. 'More', 'No', 'car', 'dolly'. There is often echolalia at this stage with the child repeating key words, mainly nouns and verbs.

**1$^1$/2 + years ' two- and three-word combinations**
These are usually an elaboration of wants or descriptions of events. 'Want more', 'Daddy gone', – followed by more varied utterances of the nature usually described as telegraphese: 'Me want it', 'All gone now', 'Bye-bye'.

**2 years – four and more words**
At this stage there is frequently processed echolalia. Phrases often used by adults are often incorporated, usually appropriately.

**2$^1$/2+ years – Linguistic explosion**
Auxiliary verbs start to be used at this stage: 'I'm gonna do it', '(It) don't go there', 'It won't go on.'
Realization that everything has a name. 'What's that?' frequently asked.

| | |
|---|---|
| (3 years) | 'Where's he going to sit?' (use of infinitive: to-) |
| | Likes to be told simple stories. |
| (3$^1$/2 years) | 'When I've finished this I'll have another one.' (Contraction of auxiliary.) |
| | Starts to learn rhymes and songs. |
| (4 years) | 'When Daddy was away at Loughborough Mummy could't win with her coffee.' (referring to game to make him eat – use of conditional tense.) |
| | Can give a short account about recent activities and events. |
| (4$^1$/2 years) | 'Why don't we play mothers and fathers?' (More complex use of interrogative.) |
| | Wants to know how and why. |
| (5 years) | 'That one looks as if it's falling.' (Analogic thought in form of similie.) |

**5 years old**
Mastery of most grammatical structures. Can make up stories.

---

The children quoted have normal non-verbal abilities and are in many ways socially proficient, travelling on their own and able to spend their pocket money sensibly. They are reliable and trustworthy, competent in most aspects of daily living. Yet their language skills are less than that of many three year-olds. By way of contrast another 14 year-old boy made up the following story:

> 'One day John was walking in the park with a dog. John's girlfriend came and met him. John asked her if they can go to Clapham station and go to the football club. John bought two tickets. When the first team scored John pushed his girlfriend and she fell over into some peoples' faces. And they dig each other. Finished.'

The use of the word 'finished' is used quite often to indicate both a hope and enquiry. It is hoped that what has been done is sufficient while at the same time being an enquiry as to whether such effort as has been made is acceptable. In books on early language development reference is often made to telegraphese. The first four children's descriptions fall into that category. Normally it is to be expected from the age of 1$^1$/2+ years onwards.

In Table 3 several examples of questions are cited. Hearing impaired children are very much less likely to ask questions and seek verbal explanations. Their language is often insufficiently structured to look at a situation, formulate their observations and deduce that additional information is needed for complete understanding. Consequently they do not so actively seek knowledge as other children do.

Some examples will make the above statements less abstruse. One child goes and sees what another child has made, perhaps some junk modelling. 'How did you do that?' Observing some actions where the end product is not apparent, 'Why are you doing that?' Both these questions show that the questioner consciously identifies gaps in his or her knowledge. Obviously it is not possible to implant questions in a child's mind. Simply getting the child by some means to ask the same questions would be to overlook all the underlying processes. Yet if a hearing impaired child is to hear, see and do the same as the other children they must be helped to observe and enquire. Sadly it is unlikely a lot can be done in an ordinary classroom setting. The best that can be aimed for is ensuring basic information is known and understood, foregoing all the usual richness and subtlety. Having said that some steps may still be taken.

## Teaching language: some classroom suggestions

### Record keeping

English is a very flexible language with a great deal of freedom in terms of word order. Such rules as there are may be broken for literary effect. James Joyce's works could not have been written in any other language. Because idiomatic expressions and usages vary from region to region, precise details cannot be given as to what should or should not be covered. This could leave teachers who have not made a special study of language in a quandary. Obviously he or she cannot be expected to embark on a detailed analysis of a hearing impaired child's language development, even if time and inclination made it a viable proposition. Yet it would be doing such a child a disservice if no attempt were made. With the introduction of the national curriculum, what was thought of as an option when making an early draft for this book will shortly become an obligation, since more comprehensive records will have to be kept for all children, as part of an ongoing assessment. Externally moderated attainment tests will form an additional part of each child's overall assessment.

The form the assessments will take in relation to the national curriculum will be based on certain assumptions, i.e. if certain recorded facts are known it can safely be assumed that others are too, e.g. once the days of the week are known and the child can count forwards and backwards, then the day following or prior to one that has been specified can be identified correctly. The framework and structure which allows retrieval of information is securely in place and makes the task easy. It is with this sort of operation that hearing impaired children are likely to be found wanting. The assumptions do not necessarily hold up.

It is suggested that any regular, obligatory record keeping is supplemented by notes detailing any deficiencies or difficulties, together with plans for remedial action. The peripatetic teacher and/or any speech therapist involved with the child should be able to assist with the latter. Since leading questions are often asked in a teaching situation to elicit information, exactly what the child says is often ignored. With the hearing impaired child it is important to listen carefully and record very accurately, including any omissions. Precisely what is said will provide an indication of what is readily understood when said to the child. That will facilitate pitching the standard of teaching at the appropriate level. As language development is almost certain to be lower than chronological age it will mean either modification at the time of presentation or additional individual input later.

Teaching new skills entails a steady progression from what is known to higher levels. The size of the steps taken increases as children get older. When children first enter school it is recognized that everything has to be explained in careful detail, letter by letter and number by number. By the time they have reached the fifth year of a secondary school the most able can understand long mathematical equations, hastily scribbled on the blackboard or complex verbal analyses. Reliance is placed on the pupils' ability to retrieve what has already been learned in order to follow what is being newly presented. Again it is the combined probabilities that topics covered previously may not have been so well learned and not so readily retrieved that have to be considered in the case of the hearing impaired child. Careful exposition, using smaller steps, is certain to be needed. This is why the majority of children who attend partially hearing units cannot cope with as wide a range of examination courses as other children of the same age. Routine teaching methods and the way they may be modified are now considered.

## Visual aids

With young children an actual object or a picture is useful. These establish a focus and help with the understanding of further information and explanations. When using visual aids remember that if the child is looking at what is being shown attention is diverted away from anything that might be said. Therefore once sufficient opportunity has been given to see what is being referred to, either obscuring it or, in the case of a picture putting it down, ensures that attention is redirected back to what is being said.

## Oral exposition

This is the most common form for introducing and presenting new information. In an ordinary mainstream situation the teacher pitches what is said at a level appropriate to the age, ability and attainments of the children in the class. If this method is used alone it is as well to check the hearing impaired child is on your wavelength. I remember taking a Religious Education lesson in a school for deaf children and asking, 'Where did Adam and Eve live?' With some perplexity a girl who had been fidgeting caught my eye and enquired, 'Where did Adam and Eve love?' (making the appropriate gesture – clasping arms about her body): this points up the importance of never underestimating the need for consistent watching by children who have to rely on lip reading.

It was in the context of Religious Education that a colleague working in another school for deaf children highlighted the need for care when using radio aids. A boy had complained his hearing aid was not working. My colleague took it to check and turned-in to a lesson in a neighbouring room. There it was clear an explanation had not been understood. A desperate cry was heard. 'It's an angel. An *angel*. A f......g *angel*.' Even specially-trained teachers of the hearing impaired can experience frustration when the most painstaking attempts fail to get a message across. In the main this is more likely to occur with children who have profound hearing losses. Shortly after I had started teaching I had failed to make one of the pupils understand. Another member of the class volunteered to help, using his knowledge of sign language to clarify the information. After about five minutes my would-be helper banged his head against the wall and exploded, 'He's so stupid!' The shared disability – hearing impairment, did not facilitate communication. Eventually I managed a satisfactory explanation, by considering in more detail *what* and *how* the necessary information could be restructured and re-presented.

## Providing context

Imagine turning on the radio or television after missing the beginning of a programme. Very often it is possible to pick up the threads after a short while. Vital pieces of information are seldom given only at the beginning and not referred to again. As the programme continues the chain of events becomes apparent. Hearing impaired children find it much harder to fill in the gaps. For them it is important to create a frame of reference and a mental set, in preparation for the sort of information to be presented. Even when this is done there is still the chance that salient features may be missed through not being heard properly. At the best of times, no matter how carefully a teacher sequences material and explains the subject matter, there is nearly always at least one child who fails to follow. The hearing impaired child is the most likely candidate for being added to that number. Most teachers will already use the methods suggested below. It is not whether they are used which counts but the consistency.

## Written words or sentences

These may be used in conjunction with other forms of visual aids or on their own. Key words or phrases, written during the course of oral exposition, serve as reminders and reinforcers. They also have the effect of providing a framework and elucidating the emerging structure.

## An integrated approach to language across the curriculum

When a new piece of information is learned it is often in an unstable form. It has been estimated that at least ten repetitions are needed for a new word to be learned by individuals with normal hearing. Those working with hearing impaired children know it is often necessary to draw attention to new words and information more often. The writing of key-words and phrases during the course of the lesson provides the opportunity for recapitulation in order to reinforce learning. It also provides a ready form of reference for inclusion in other settings where appropriate. Recall after a couple of days and then a week later are helpful. In practice this is what is done with homework at secondary school. The teacher gives the lesson. Some individual work is usually done immediately. Homework is set, marked and the main points dealt with together with any omissions at a later stage. Periodic tests help to revive the knowledge and facilitate its recall. Hearing impaired children need such structuring of what is to be learned to promote long-term memory. Mathematical terms, because they are abstract in nature, even though they are often illustrated in practical ways, also need to be reinforced in a variety of ways and this can be done in the normal course of events, e.g. instead of only saying, 'Give out the . . .', elaborate. Point out that there is enough material for one each, between two, per table, etc., and it will be divided up in that way. It is only by such means that the hearing impaired child is likely to get sufficient reinforcement, through many repetitions to learn both the meanings and the associated language structures.

These needs may look more than a classroom teacher could undertake. The national curriculum could be helpful. In the Interim Report, Design and Technology Group it is stated,

> Design and technological activities in a range of contexts is important not only to encourage pupils' motivation for learning, but also to ensure for them a balanced experience of the use of different resources of knowledge and skills and of the appraisal of constraints (p. 8; 1.18).

and

> most primary and secondary schools will already be providing some experience of design and technological activity for their pupils, though this will not always be formally recognized and designated as such . . . we see our attainment targets and programmes of study offering a

clear and firm framework for existing practice in these and related curriculum areas (p. 9; 1.20).

The point being made is that there must be a more formal structure to link dis-
parate parts of the core and foundation subjects. Once this is established it
should make integration easier to accomplish in terms of language.

## Identification of words, phrases and grammatical structures to be learned

When children have had a painting lesson they readily understand that they
*must* wash their hands. *Must* and *mustn't* are easily conveyed. Deaf people who
use sign language have a specific sign for it. 'You should wash your hands,
now,' has nearly the same meaning, but is nowhere near so easily understood
by hearing impaired children, as it does not contain the same element of com-
pulsion. Every young child has had the experience of being made to do something. It serves to reinforce the meaning of *must*. Thereafter the use of an
equivalent word is readily understood. It should not be assumed hearing impaired children are so familiar or understand so readily such varied ways of
speaking.

Children are usually informed when it is nearly time to finish an activity
and start clearing away. This can be done in a large variety of ways: 'You've
got another five minutes,' 'It's nearly time to stop,' 'Start finishing off now,'
'You should get ready to stop soon.' These are all fairly abstract statements,
intended to create a mental set. For the hearing impaired child it is particularly important to ensure the message is understood. The opportunity should be
taken in a variety of settings to use the same terminology. With the example
of painting or craft work the practical aspects help to make the meaning clear.
In a test situation or when engaged in a written exercise, estimating time is less
easy. When recapitulating a series of instruction it is easy to incorporate *should*.
'First you should ... then you should ...' etc.

There will be other times when the negative forms are used, *mustn't* and
*shouldn't*. Remember that when the contracted form is used it is almost indistinguishable from the instruction to do. Try saying both. Because of where the
tongue finishes up 'n't' almost gets lost, especially for anyone lip reading. The
eye is nowhere near as good as the ear in perceiving subtleties of this kind. So
although it is necessary to teach the use of contractions, when giving instructions it is helpful to use the full form for negatives to avoid confusion.

## Role play

A simple statement such as, 'John was not feeling well yesterday,' seems so obvious as not to require any further attention. Yet it is not so easily understood
as, 'John was ill.' The actual feeling of objects and role playing may be required
to make the meaning understood. In PE the children could be asked to walk

as if feeling tired, to push out their chests and smile as when feeling happy. At secondary level although the strategies given above can be used it is not so easy to use similar structures in different subject settings. Most schools have a Special Needs Department to help children with reading difficulties. The staff there will be familiar with the different syllabi in order to incorporate the subject content with their support teaching. This puts them in a good position to make suggestions for any hearing impaired child.

# 5   Speech and Language – The Specifics

The need to integrate all the work done with hearing impaired children is a constantly recurring theme on which variations are played. This point has been appreciated in respect of other children too, as the quotations from the national curriculum indicated (p. 56). It was emphasized in Chapter 4 how the varying amounts of diminished auditory experience imbalances the whole learning process to some degree. Consequently levels of understanding must be constantly checked and coordinated with efforts to enrich both vocabulary and knowledge of other linguistic structures. This naturally applies to the interlinked fields of reading, writing and spelling. The areas to which special attention should be paid can be highlighted within the context of normal practices. Table 4 presents an overview of these. More details are given in Appendix B which can serve as an *aide memoire*.

**Table 4: Aims and approaches for teaching literacy and oracy**

| *Aims* | | | |
|---|---|---|---|
| *Speaking* | *Listening* | *Reading* | *Writing* |
| To provide the opportunity to develop oral skills of communication and express thoughts fluently | To develop the abiliy to listen with under-standing, enjoyment and discernment | To encourage and develop a desire to read | To develop the ability to express in writing original ideas |
| *Skills and activities* | | | |
| Articulation<br>Making statements<br>Asking questions<br>Describing<br>Narrating<br>Speaking effectively in public | Discernment of:<br>intonation<br>punctuation<br><br>Stories, poems and rhymes<br>Retelling<br>Learning by heart<br><br>Comprehension exercises<br><br>Increasing listening span<br><br>Discrimination of character<br><br>**Musical instruments**<br><br>Identification of:<br>(1) source, (2) direction, (3) quality, (4) duration, (5) pitch | Whole word recognition<br>Phonics<br>Use of context<br><br>Reading silently<br><br>Introduction to library<br><br>(1) Use of reference books<br>(2) Selection of data | Gross motor skills<br>Fine hand control<br><br>Use of tools<br><br>Punctuation<br><br>Spelling<br><br>Homophones<br><br>Advanced grammar<br><br>Style |

Since the fields indicated by Table 4 are so broad only those areas related to sounds, music and speaking will be dealt with in this chapter. In order to provide a framework they are slotted into sections. The interconnected and overlapping nature of the topics means that dealing with certain variables in one section as opposed to another may appear arbitrary. This is inevitable. There are virtually endless ways in which the same data can be reorganized and reclassified into sets and subsets.

## Breath control and articulation

The clarify of hearing impaired children's speech is largely determined by the nature and degree of their hearing loss. Experienced teachers of hearing impaired children can in most cases specify these features fairly accurately from just listening. This applies as much to children who wear hearing aids as those that do not. The links between what is heard and what is said is very precise, due to the regulatory role auditory feedback plays on the control of speech musculature. This should not be taken to mean that there is nothing productive to be done. Speech practice might not result in major improvements in clarity, certainly not in the short term, but it is likely to lead to a better ability to make sense of what is heard, especially spoken language. A further benefit later is a better ability to use a phonic attack, when necessary, by making them aware of speech sounds and the segmentation of words.

The almost exclusive reliance on hearing aids to make up for deficits has led to underlying processes being ignored in some settings. A one-time very influential figure in the training of teachers of the deaf perhaps did one of the greatest disservices to hearing impaired children by stating, 'A deaf child is a normal child who cannot hear.' This is patently misleading and untrue. The deprivation of the full range of auditory experiences affects virtually every aspect of daily life, calling for every effort to be made to minimise adverse effects in every area that can be identified.

It is not expected that the non-specialist should do the work of either a teacher of the hearing impaired or a speech therapist, but there are activities which can be undertaken without specialist knowledge or training. First, there are the purely instrumental aspects of speech. To speak at all there must be a flow of air through the speech mechanisms. The flow has to be precisely and intricately controlled. Hearing impaired children often do not have good breath control, for reasons given earlier. Improvement can be promoted by specific exercises. These are in no way complicated and can be incorporated into any session involving physical exercise. One of the simplest is to have the children standing, legs slightly apart, with hands on hips; first breathing in deeply, through the nose, letting the shoulders droop slightly, then breathing out slowly through the mouth. With young children breathing out can be to the count of two or three, the count being extended for older children, to about ten eventually, once sufficient control is achieved. This particular exercise should not be repeated too frequently without a break, otherwise some children may feel dizzy. Instead of simply breathing out the children can hum or make any speech sounds, for example, continuous, open vowel sounds or punctuated ones (pah, pah, pah, pah), possibly in time with the teacher's count. Pretending to toss the sounds forwards, upwards and downwards adds another dimension.

There are two rather old-fashioned methods which at one time formed part of a battery of articulation exercises. The empirical way in which they were devised before being used and refined over the years, means they are still valid ways of teaching breath control to children with hearing losses. The first consists of carefully controlling the stream of breath to vary the angle to which a candle flame is blown. Games and activities such as blow football and blow-painting serve a similar function, but with less precision. Blowing bubbles is a perennial pastime commonly used for the same ends. Although not strictly speaking a game, blowing over the curve of a piece of thin paper (about 6 x 6 inches) held between finger and thumb makes the whole piece rise. This incidentally is used to illustrate aerodynamic principles in physics. Children are likely to spontaneously compete to see who could keep the paper up longest. The other method, now ignored, involves puffing off little pieces of tissue paper from the back of the hand when making plosive and fricative sounds (b, p, k, t, d, s, sh). Such methods have tended to pass into disuse with the advent of electronic devices. The drawback of a display on monitor screens is that it relies solely on visual feedback, making no use of other senses to reinforce each other as in the case of the methods described, i.e. kinaesthesis, proprioception, tactile and visual.

At one time I lived in a flat below Margaret Price, before she became an internationally renowned operatic star. One weekend she was rehearsing her part in the Verdi *Requiem*, which at one point requires a dramatic leap to a very demanding top note. The accompaniment played. She started and missed. Again and again and again this was repeated – throughout the whole of one Saturday. She started again the following Sunday morning and towards noon achieved perfection. This is mentioned as an outstanding example of the need of even the most highly skilled for continuous practice. That those who lack the essential sense for acquiring normal articulation automatically should be given consistent practice follows without further comment.

Wind instruments provide a natural progression to further refinement of breath control. Any wind instrument can be used of course, but in practice the melodica is most likely to be the one of choice. It produces a loud sound and is fairly simple to control. At any one time a specific skill will form the focus, but it is seldom that other features will be of no account. Volume control is naturally associated with any sound production. The control developed by the activities listed above help when modulation of the voice is called for. Recitation of nursery rhymes at an early stage, poems and songs later, provide good opportunities for increasing awareness of loudness or softness to accentuate meaning and expressiveness, along with changes in pitch. Once the words have been well learned attention is freed to be focused on this kind of refinement.

The work done in relation to speaking, namely intonation, pauses, etc., are vital in relationship to later written work, when basic punctuation is taught. Unless the features to be transcribed are well established in the child's repertoire they will simply remain meaningless symbols on the page, certain to be forgotten in creative writing, even if used correctly in workbook exercises. It is more important for hearing impaired children to carefully build up skills stage by stage. This is common practice in other areas such as either concentrating on the content of what is written or the neatness of the writing. In the early stages few children can do both.

The need for the teacher to speak distinctly has already been mentioned. Because hearing impaired children may not hear all speech sounds clearly, especially those with ski-slope hearing losses, they omit the sounds they cannot hear when speaking themselves. This can make it difficult for others to understand what they are saying. If nothing is done to draw attention to defective articulation not only will improvements fail to occur but reading and spelling will be harder to learn, due to an even greater than usual lack of correspondence between what is said and seen. Some published advice states that teachers should just talk normally to hearing impaired children. This does not seem to make sense when normal developmental patterns are considered. First children notice gross differences. Only after a great deal of experience and practice are finer and finer details heeded. Therefore some exaggeration can be helpful, especially when it is necessary to emphasise features the child is evidently unaware of. At meetings of adults with a profound hearing loss 'lip speakers' are often employed. They often simplify what is being said and project the information by using greatly exaggerated lip, tongue and facial movements. To what extent the exaggeration they use is necessary or desirable will depend on individual children's need to lip read and how far the speaker is from them. Some classrooms are large and in a gymnasium or on the sports field the distances involved will certainly be too great most of the time to see clearly what is said if normal speech patterns are employed.

There are certain categories of words that are likely to cause confusion, homophones in particular. Hearing impaired children are less able to make use of context in order to automatically select the appropriate meaning. Naturally no matter what the clarity of the visual pattern, it is the combination of sound and context that is important. Plurals and contractions may also present difficulties. Specialized vocabulary tends to be polysyllabic as exemplified by that used in connection with punctuation, for example (PunCTuaTIOn/aPoSTroPHE/QUeSTion). This makes it more difficult to discriminate accurately initially and therefore to memorise. There are also many high frequency sounds, depicted by capital letters. But that is true for so many words. Therein lies the trouble.

## Sounds

In this section the nature of sound, environmental sounds and topic work that could arise from them are dealt with first. This leads on to some musical activities non-music specialists could confidently undertake. Everyday sounds have musical qualities, which have inspired composers to make references to them, as in Beethoven's *Pastoral Symphony*. Nothing so ambitious is envisaged for the classroom, but the sounds about us are fascinating and exciting in their own right and worthy of exploitation in an educational setting.

### The nature of sound

The pure tones used for audiometry each consist of just one frequency and lack any kind of warmth. Naturally occurring sounds are never pure tones. It is the mixture of harmonics that distinguishes one person's voice from another and creates the characteristic, attractive qualities of different instruments. Some sounds travel better than others. Long waves go further than short waves, the higher pitched ones. The latter have less energy and can only be heard over shorter distances. Since some consonants (s, k, f, t, etc.) consist mainly of the higher frequencies in the speech range they fade away to almost nothing in large rooms and certainly in school halls. Hence the question often asked by speakers, 'Can you hear me at the back?' The sometimes shouted, 'No', shows this not to be true, but it does signify the speaker is talking too quietly for easy listening.

Sound, unlike light can go round corners, which makes environmental sounds bathe us almost equally whether we are facing the source or not. When listening to the radio we are free to move. This makes it a less demanding occupation than watching television, where watching is obligatory, if the programme is to be followed. Comparatively speaking, children with normal hearing are in the position of radio listeners, hearing impaired children have to be more attentive, looking consistently as well as listening. This imposes an unnatural strain. Consequently they may well appear to have a shorter attention span than the others. The greater effort required to watch unremittingly uses up part of the total (mental) energy available. A hearing impaired child cannot be expected to 'listen' for such prolonged periods as normally hearing ones who do not have to make the same simultaneously concentrated effort.

Straining to make full use of one sense, dulls the others. Looking intently leads to sounds being overlooked and vice versa. Because people with normal sight and hearing are seldom in that situation it is necessary to state the obvious. On one occasion I was talking about this to a group which included a congenitally deaf social worker. He interrupted to get confirmation from the others that a tennis ball really did make a swishing sound as it went through the air. So no apology is made for mentioning what is self-evident to people with normal hearing, such as the fact each one of us is in the centre of our own auditory environment. We just accept without a second thought the way environmental sounds keep us constantly in touch with what is happening all around. There is no reason to take notice. The failure to do so could mean missed opportunities for alerting hearing impaired children to information of significance if they are to derive the fullest and deepest understanding of the normal everyday events. Environmental sounds govern a variety of behaviours incidentally as well as keeping us in touch with what is happening all around. The sound of the wind howling outside might prompt a remark such as, 'Brr! Listen to that. I'm glad I'm inside in the warm', thereby stimulating a social interaction. We are struck by the quietness in libraries and places of worship and behave accordingly. Young children respond quickly to the suggestion they keep their mouths closed while eating, avoiding lip-smacking sounds or noisily sucking up the last drops through a straw. Similarly it is seldom necessary to tell children not to shuffle their feet along. Depending on the degree of hearing loss such comments may have to be made to hearing-impaired children.

Children with a big hearing loss derive pleasure from the sensations like scraping the soles of their shoes. Even people with normal hearing enjoy scuffing their feet through drifts of leaves in a forest. With some of the other sounds referred to there may be similar pleasure. To stop a child with normal hearing from including pleasurable but socially unacceptable noises in their everyday repertoire, imposes no hardship. The same must apply to the hearing impaired. They will have sufficient difficulty in life, without being burdened by habits others find disagreeable.

Nearby sounds have a wider range of frequencies than distant ones. This gives them a sharpness which acts as a clue to how far away the source of the sound is. Enough has already been said about high-frequency hearing losses to make it plain how they interfere with this phenomenon. The changes in the loudness and clarity of sounds can serve as a warning. Babies often look about when they hear footsteps. This alerts them and avoids their being startled. Babies who have a significant hearing loss are not so protected.

A number of environmental sounds are listed below, every one familiar. Each could be described baldly in terms of its physical characteristics, but they have personally relevant associations. It is those social connotations that enhance interest in them. The sounds associated with the bathroom can be of desperate interest if the room is occupied by another member of the family and an urgent call of nature has to be answered by the one waiting outside. Sounds emanating from the kitchen can excite gastric juices and heighten pangs of hunger.

The selection of sounds listed in Table 5 highlight the fact we are probably living in a more informative auditory environment than at any other period in history. In our daily life it is possible to monitor the activities of our own homes by listening. How many people have experienced the aggravating wait for a toilet cistern to refill, or shrieked at the hiss and splutter of an overflowing saucepan? Many hearing impaired children may not hear such sounds or only hear them in such a distorted way as not to be able to interpret them ac-

**Table 5: Socially-informative sounds**

---

*Domestic*

| | |
|---|---|
| Bathroom | Water: running into the basin; down the plug-hole; flushing the WC; the cistern refilling; splashing droplets as a flannel is rung out; brushing nails and teeth; turning lock; buzz of fluorescent tube. |
| Kitchen | Hiss of gas; water heating up; drinks fizzing; saucepans boiling over; food frying; potatoes being scraped; chopping vegetables; packets being opened; mechanical aids (grinders, blenders, mixers etc.) |
| Living-room | Curtains being drawn; laying table; clink of crockery; sounds accompanying meals; rustle of paper and magazines being read; clocks; sliding doors; click of catches; turning handles; post delivery; doorbell; vacuum cleaner. |
| Garden | Digging; hoeing; raking; sieving; pruning; burning refuse; watering. |

*General*

| | |
|---|---|
| Weather | Wind; rain; rustling leaves; thunder. |
| Animals | Cats; dogs; horses; birds; etc. |
| Traffic | Cars, motor-bikes, lorries; taxis; sirens; aeroplanes; milk-floats; bells; hooters; swish of tyres; screech of brakes; beeping at traffic lights for blind people; refuse disposal collection. |

| | |
|---|---|
| *Shopping* | Announcements; 'musak'; electronic scanner; till; theft alarm; ice-cream van. |

| | |
|---|---|
| *Recreational* | Bands; buskers; discos; concerts. |

---

curately. Another important point to remember is that a hearing aid takes away a good sense of direction. It interferes with the normal functioning of the ears. Even if two are worn location of sound is very poor. In the section on the ear mention was made of the two tiny muscles in the middle ear. Apart from affecting the tension of the ear to make it more sensitive to high frequency sounds they also help with the location of sound. A slight hearing loss, especially one caused by glue ears, impairs this ability. Children so affected look about more than others, sometimes creating a spurious impression of brightness by their constant interest in all that is going on around.

Whether the term *auditory training* has any meaning was at one time discussed as heatedly by those who taught the deaf as, 'How many angels can dance on a pin-head?' was by medieval monks. It is certainly possible to teach children to discriminate between certain sounds. A start can be made in a nonthreatening way in a musical setting, hence the presentation at this point. It is part of an accepted behaviour pattern to keep quiet and concentrate on the music which makes music lessons a good setting for repeated practice to develop auditory discrimination. The following features may be illustrated. The first two are often used in the form of a game at pre-school level, by peripatetic teachers.

1    *Identification* – What made the sound?


2    *Location* – (Two or more children can be positioned with the same instrument and without looking the other children have to identify which one has made the sound.)


3    *Pitch* – Was the sound high or low? (Intermediate can be added later.)


4    *Loudness* – Was the sound loud or soft?


5    *Quality* – Was the sound pleasant or unpleasant? There is likely to be disagreement about certain sounds.


With this five-way classification the children will eventually be abe to give a complete description of what instrument was played where, how loudly, at what pitch and whether it was agreeable or disagreeable. To be able to do this the various characteristics must be already familiar. How many can be described will depend on the age and memory span of the children. The relevant information has to be held in mind while translated into spoken language. Anyone who has not worked with disabled children is likely to be unaware of the amount of effort involved in exerting conscious control over clarity of speech. This observation applies more to children having significant losses of course, but it is important since concentrating on the mechanics of speech diminishes the capacity left for remembering. The other factor affecting accuracy of report will be the clarity with which each of the variables registered in the first place. This leads to uncertainty and in turn a lack of assurance. Constant doubts have a debilitating effect. The upshot of all these interacting variables is that by and large the hearing impaired child will manage one item less than the average for the class at any given stage. For the more severely hearing impaired an even lower comparative level may be expected.

Once some practice has been given in a musical setting, analysis of environmental sounds emerges quite naturally. There are some loud ones which are certain to be heard, while others like the whine of a gnat, or the rustle of tissue paper may never be. Some sounds, especially at nursery stage, help to develop motor skills. The most common are encountered in the following activities.

WATERPLAY

When playing with water the splashing is evident. By listening intently can the child tell the following: Is the water being splashed or poured in a continuous stream? The sound made when a container is being filled changes as the air is displaced. Can the child tell how full a given container is by listening and detect the abrupt change of sound when it is about to overflow, taking appropriate action if necessary?

SANDTRAY

Can the child hear dry sand as it swishes through a funnel and detect the following? The change of tone as a bucket packed with damp sand is tapped and the moulded sand falls free – indicating the right time to remove the container? Most children learn to identify when this happens without its being pointed out. Hearing impaired children tend to miss clues of this subtlety.

CUTTING AND SAWING

Just before wood is cut through completely the changed pitch of the sound made forewarns it is nearly severed. This helps to regulate our movements, prompting care to avoid a ragged finish. To some extent the same is true when cutting paper and card. It is only with the last snip that the click of the blades alters as they are completely freed. The auditory signal confirms the completion of the action and serves as a reward for correct programming – on most occasions. It will now be evident how the development of motor skills is assisted by hearing and why the teacher of a hearing impaired child should draw attention to them, explaining the process clearly. Topic work related to environmental sounds calls for tape-recordings and a host of other activities. By using the sounds made as a starting point other features connected with natural phenomena can be dealt with. In addition to being of value to the whole class this will help the hearing impaired child specifically, expanding understanding of associations and relationships. In most instances any work undertaken will reveal the higher order practical skills of the children with normal hearing, as well as their more extensive vocabulary. Some topics are suggested below.

## Level 1 (5+ years old) – Where have you heard water?

The likely answers will include: turning on taps; filling a bowl, bath or basin; water running away; rain; the sea-shore; a waterfall; a stream; water boiling; splashing in a pool; the plop when a fish jumps out. The accounts and onomatopoeic words used will give an indication of the range of an average child's knowledge. During the course of any individual work with the hearing impaired child whether the most commonly mentioned facts are known can be checked and if not, specifically taught. Work of this kind lends itself to reinforcement in music. The swishing of brushes on cymbals and drums makes a good accompaniment for flowing movements; the tinkling glockenspiel suggests rain drops and a rising drum-roll with the final thump as the waves crash down.

## *Level 2 (7+ years old) – What have you heard opened?*

In many ways this seems similar to Level 1, but it is different in nature because of its specificity and the need for an ability to perceive relationships. Some quite sophisticated examples could crop up: slitting (tearing) open an envelope; a door; a screw-top bottle; a corked bottle; a can of drink; unwrapping a parcel; a box; a car boot; a window (sash type); a drawer; a new shop (by a celebrity); a soap packet; a tin, etc. Children of this age are quite likely to volunteer things which do not have any associated sounds, such as mouth and eyes. By this stage children can usually categorize, but it may be very difficult to describe the sounds in such a way as to group them. It might be worth the effort. In the main the sorts of sounds referred to are not so often commented upon as those connected with water, hence the dearth of appropriate adjectives.

## *Level 3 (9+ years old) – Domestic sounds*

Some or all of the sounds listed above may be elicited, plus a few more that are unflattering to other members of the family, e.g. snoring and eructations. At this age children tend to be good observers and to have the openness to talk about what they have seen and heard. The hearing impaired child's lesser awareness of sound related events and poorer ability to describe them will be more apparent by now. The wide variations between children makes it impossible to pin-point the deficits for any one individual. Comparisons with the local population, specifically other members of the class are the most reliable guide.

## *Level 4 (11+) – Noise pollution*

At this age children are able to think in abstract terms. The ability to do so starts to emerge at about the age of eight and is normally well developed by the time children transfer to secondary school. It is probable most members of the class will be able to identify the sorts of sounds which are regarded as polluting our environment and give reasons why they are undesirable. Many will have noticed men using pneumatic drills wear ear-protectors. The hearing impaired child will doubtless get the idea that unpleasant, maybe loud noises are being mentioned, but the concept of pollution is likely to be hazy. This could be checked by asking about air or water pollution. The majority of the children in the class would be expected to come up with some ideas about what pollutes. In the event of the hearing impaired child obviously not understanding it can be explained at the simpler level of loud noises being unpleasant and upsetting people, which is why they should be stopped wherever possible. This is obviously not the fundamental concept that it is intended to convey, but it may well be as close as it is possible to get. Ideally continuous monitoring and assessment of a hearing impaired child's progress is called for.

In practice, as one of a class of thirty or more children, the amount of time available is limited.

It is not intended to detail all the areas that might be covered by such topics since the core curriculum documents for English, Mathematics, Science and Design and Technology each specify in their own way how topics such as these may be used to stimulate understanding of the separate disciplines. An indication in respect of one might be a helpful focus, however. With domestic sounds the algebraic relationships might be identified in terms of whether they are generated by machinery, peoples' actions or noises made by the individuals themselves. The noise level of equipment could be converted into statistical data and plotted on a graph. This would lead on to a later topic, in which more precise measurements could be made with a sound-level meter. The noises made by individuals relate to talking, digestive sounds, laughing, sighing, snoring, etc. Biology is encompassed in this way. Tape recorders could be used for doors shutting, hinges squeaking, creaks caused by the warming up of pipes in the central heating. Each and every aspect has its own vocabulary, together with an appropriate explanation. The teaching and analysis will serve to link information in a way that is helpful to hearing impaired children, whilst developing the skills needed for standardized assessment tasks.

When children are in their last year of primary school staff often become anxious about whether a child will be able to cope in secondary school and urgent to obtain extra help. Should the child be markedly below the level of other members of the class the possibility of making a Statement of Special Educational Need should be mooted, if it has not already been done. Unless extra individual teaching is arranged, or alternatively transfer to a secondary school in which a partially hearing unit is housed, there will be a further steady falling behind. As the National Curriculum is constructed in the form of a continuum there should not be such an abrupt change as is presently the case, though as is noted in the Mathematics proposals,

> the framework is broad enough to accommodate a range of approaches to meeting individual pupil needs. However, it is most unlikely that a scheme of work within this framework that is designed for the majority will be satisfactory for those with special needs. For example, a pupil aged 14 whose mathematical attainment is judged to be that of an average 7 year old will need a different teaching programme and approach from a 14 year old of average attainment (p. 89; 10.31).

## Music

Enjoyment of music appears to be a fundamental characteristic of human beings. Given the opportunity, people who claim not to be able to sing a note join in enthusiastically with a sing-song. Fortunately most young children do not have a well developed critical faculty and are quite happy to listen to an adult. A good voice is not essential, provided reasonable intonation can be managed.

## Instruments

In schools with a specialist music teacher, other teachers tend to be coy about using instruments. There are a range which can be used, even by those without any formal training. They will be dealt with later.

### Radio, tapes and discs

These are the most accessible sources of music, but their big drawback for hearing impaired children is not being visible or tangible and unless they are played very loudly they do not have the same immediacy as real instruments. As everyone knows the quality of music is very different in a live performance. A brass band, accompanied by a big bass drum wallops the gut, strikes the ear and invites the whole body to swing along. With quieter music the sensations received by other parts of the body are less noticeable, but they do occur, making live music preferable every time.

## Activities to develop awareness of sound and motor skills

### Musical

For the non-specialist it is probable that only percussion instruments will be used: drums; tambourines; maracas; blocks; chime-bars; cymbals; glockenspiel; triangle; xylophone, etc. To begin the children's exploration should be non-directed, allowing them to find out for themselves how many ways sounds can be produced. It is important not to stifle natural curiosity and inventiveness, otherwise some approaches may be overlooked, e.g. stroking the skin of a (good quality) tambourine to make a much more gentle and mysterious sound than the customary banging and jingling. A whole range of percussion instruments with serrations can be voiced by stick or thumb-nail to make either discrete clicks or a zipping sound. If xylophones and glockenspiels are used removing the relevant chimes to leave the pentatonic scale avoids cacophony. Once instruments have been explored and the children have discovered what they can do themselves, they are naturally interested in what else can be achieved. Rhythmic work is a natural starting point. Initially some rhythms will have to be demonstrated. Once the children have got the hang of rhythm, members of the class can be invited to make them up for the others to copy. A variant is for the children to take turns, rather like passing the parcel. Instead of an object the rhythm is passed on. This is repeated by the recipient, but a different one is passed on. If a child is unable to think of a different rhythm the proceedings should not be held up. Another variation is to pretend a question is being asked and the next child has to reply, e.g. 'slow quick/slow/quick quick?' (What are/you/doing?) 'slow quick/quick/slow (making a cake). The more adept may well use variations in loudness as a substitute for pitch. For young children it is probably best to suggest they actually think of a question, ask it and then tap the rhythm. The reply can be given in the same way. After a bit of practice the verbal part can be omitted. This sort of activity is good for the hearing impaired child as it does not make great demands on linguistic ability, while emphasizing the underlying rhythms of speech.

The voice is the most readily available instrument and the one that needs most practice. Although la-la is the most familiar for rhythmic work, any combination of consonant/vowel may be used. Once rhythms and melodic line are imitated readily it is time to move on and incorporate movement, first clapping, then hopping and stepping. Eventually a combination of voice, movement and use of portable percussion instrument is the goal. Before attempting such combinations each skill must be well established. This is why the voice and body movements are paired to begin with. Each additional activity imposes a greater load on what can be remembered and performed simultaneously. Practice (making the activity second nature in a sense) has the effect of reducing the amount of central capacity devoted to performance, enabling a variety of simultaneous actions.

The suggested rhythms to be tapped out for questions and answers above did not match the spoken form very closely. Visual notation can make the correspondence closer. With formal musical notation this is done by means of the breve, the semi-breve, etc. Dashes of different lengths can be used instead, with oblique strokes to indicate groups. Apart from the direct relevance to the musical activity a reading sub-skill is practised, i.e. following along the line from left to right. The hearing impaired child is sure to find these activities hard because s/he only receives a partial signal. There tends to be a fairly direct correlation between degree of hearing loss and level of skill, resulting in poor rhythmic skills and an inability to sing in tune. The visual cues help draw attention to variations which may not be so apparent through hearing.

As far as the normal musical curriculum is concerned the hearing impaired child will naturally be expected to take part in singing and the learning of instruments, unless the hearing loss is so great as to prevent pitch control of the voice and discrimination of the entire range of any given instrument. This is not to say he or she should be forbidden from making an attempt if so inclined.

## Implications for classroom organization

Sound travels round corners. Light does not. To see what is said the view must be unobstructed, the reason for a horse-shoe arrangement of desks in many schools for the 'deaf' and partially hearing units, so every child can see all the others. The way most mainstream classrooms are organized nowadays means that it is often virtually impossible for hearing impaired children to see everyone else. It is important to be aware of the limitations this imposes on hearing impaired children for supplementing what they cannot hear with lip reading. Therefore, whenever possible children engaged in any group activity should be arranged in a circle or similar configuration so all are visible to each other. With the sorts of activities and topic work described above this should not be too difficult. To what extent it is possible at other times will depend on local circumstances.

# 6  Reading, Writing and Associated Activities

This Chapter is in effect a continuation of the last and still relates to Table 4: the activities described are interlinked with those in Chapter 5. The justification for this is that no opportunity should be missed to illustrate how care should be taken to avoid misunderstanding by omitting what may seem an irrelevant detail.

## Reading and writing 'attack skills'

Initial reading and writing 'attack skills' are normally taught to children with profound hearing losses as early as two years, the age at which many embark on their formal education, within the normal constraints of nursery education. Since one of the first things learned is one's own name, this and the names of other children in the class are stuck on the backs of chairs. This serves to establish personal identity, the identity of others and some idea of personal possession. By saying the child's name and pointing to the name on the chair, what is said and what is written is associated. The child is also encouraged to speak its own name and that of classmates. A further activity is tracing over the letters with a finger. Since tactile and kinaesthetic sensations are so helpful in reinforcing the other senses, a similar procedure can be adopted with many objects in the classroom. To permit the children to do this the labels must be at a suitable height. Simply labelling without direct involvement results in what is written being disregarded and no more heeded than the wallpaper.

I suspect the majority of teachers in nursery and infant schools will respond to the above suggestions by thinking that that's alright then. It is already our practice. Like everything else it is not merely a question of whether it is done, but with what frequency and consistency. The intention of the many repetitions is to produce a dialectical leap whereby quantitive accumulation leads to qualitative changes, in this case a change from familiarity to understanding and spontaneous usage. For children with all their senses, the combination of inputs results in much quicker learning, obviating the need for what must be beginning to seem an obsessional emphasis on repetition and repeated reinforcement. As indicated in the preface there will be some exceptions and some very bright hearing impaired children will cope successfully without.

One teenager I assessed had managed up to the end of the fifth form of a Grammar School. The extra demands made in the Sixth Form, once he embarked on A Level examinations meant he no longer could. At that stage he transferred to a school with a partially hearing unit and given the extra language support needed, even at that advanced level, he succeeded. This particular case has been mentioned as there does seem to have been a great deal of concentration on early years. It serves to illustrate the necessity for vigilance at every stage. The fact that everyday conversations are adequate should not be allowed to mask difficulties with higher order thinking processes, or lead to a facile ascription of generally low abilities as being the root cause for lack of success.

The use of pictures and visual aids was mentioned in relation to the use of hearing aids and general classroom strategies. Ideally any pictures or other visual aids should only be displayed when they are to be used directly. If they are merely put up to decorate the walls *habituation* will ensue. This is the process by which often repeated stimuli come to be ignored. Novelty catches the attention. Hearing impaired children often find it difficult to sustain attention, so any stimulus that catches it should not be squandered. Black and white photographs from newspapers present information with stark clarity, more dramatically than illustrations and there is usually much detail, often omitted from pictures in story books. In every nursery and infant school there are numerous introductory books that defy conversation. The pictures do not tell a story and often bear little relationship to any text. The stated aim in Table 6 is to encourage and develop a desire to read. Leafing through picture books is a pastime. Many children have had experience of it before entering school. Articulate children have been known to express dissatisfaction at being expected to play instead of learning.

Each school has its own reading scheme, usually consisting of one or more series of readers and work-books. Additional reading material, suited to the stage reached by any individual child, is typically available. Particular schemes favoured by some schools for the hearing impaired and partially hearing units are listed in the bibliography. Just two are worthy of special mention, since they fulfil fairly specific functions. The first of these is *Stories in Pictures*, by John Goodall. They contain a wealth of detail and make apparent the events depicted in dynamic terms, so that each picture does provide a talking point. There are of course plenty of other materials which portray many varied activities, e.g. a picture of the countryside with children climbing, birds flying, ducks swimming, etc. These can be used, especially at the earlier stages, but the questions they provoke and the answers elicited tend to be very limited. The Goodall books add a time dimension, partly by the use of flaps which when turned show before and after. The other series is the *Mirror Books*, published by André Deutsch. The basic idea is a very simple one. By suitably positioning the mirror on each page the reflection completes the picture. But contrasts and other relationships are highlighted, e.g. a sad face and a smiling one. These are very familiar already. The action of placing the mirror adds a sparkle. The contents are very varied and are also used to illustrate certain mathematical concepts, as well as linguistic ones.

The approaches to teaching reading used in special schools are virtually the same as in others. Again it is a question of degree. A continuous feature of the teaching is the writing up of any keywords and phrases, so that reading and writing are not separate activities, but inextricably linked with listening and speaking. Another difference is sitting opposite, instead of next to, so the child can look up directly and see what the teacher says as well as making any use

73

of hearing. Even with this very much greater emphasis on reading and writing skills, the majority of hearing impaired children still lag behind their peers. The reasons were given in Chapter 4. A reminder is given in the next section, of steps to encourage language development insofar as it relates to reading.

## Asking questions, interactionary verbal abilities

Hearing impaired children's ability to ask questions is often delayed. Most children ask lots of questions. Some of the most common are: 'What are you doing? How do you do that? Why are you doing it? Can I have a go? Do you know . . . ? When are we going? Is the minute up yet?'

By questioning children elicit a lot of information and often follow up one question with another, thereby prompting further verbal interaction. Their command of language is sufficiently developed to formulate questions in a variety of ways. Typically the enquiries are framed to elicit answers suited to their level of understanding. One of the questions listed above is quite sophisticated. 'Do you know?' is often a way of getting someone else to ask the questioner a question, the expectation being that the one addressed does not know. In English we do not signal what answer we expect from the way in which we formulate a question, as is done in Latin. There, three forms are used depending on whether a yes or a no answer is anticipated or if it is a straightforward request for information. In English we can signal what we think the answer should be by intonation, as when a child thought to be greedy is asked, 'Do you want *another* piece of cake?' It is very seldom a hearing impaired child will ask a question with this degree of subtlety and sophistication. As all the many question forms that children use cannot be listed, a record should be made of the questions other children ask. Armed with that information teaching situations can be devised wherein the hearing impaired pupil may learn both the form of the question and be encouraged to use it. This will lead to some rather stilted situations at times, but it is unavoidable. Relying entirely on natural processes does not work.

The speaking effectively in public listed in Table 5 is not in practice the ultimate stage. Hearing impaired children, either because their speech is not clear, and/or they have insufficient language to express themselves fluently may easily be deterred from making contributions if continually asked to repeat or clarify what they have said. If it is the practice to encourage children to stand up and tell others little items of news or to show a piece of work and talk about it, some prior coaching of the hearing impaired child is helpful. By appropriate positioning lip read prompts can be given. This would apply especially if it takes place in a hall as part of an assembly. When hearing is normal it is possible to gauge how loudly one is talking by the echo. A hearing aid confuses this feedback. By turning it down slightly so that the child has to speak more loudly to hear himself or herself at the accustomed volume, projection might be encouraged. When a paradoxical affect might be encountered it will be necessary to turn the volume up. The same principle will apply to choral work. As ever despite generalizations each child has to be treated according to his or her own lights.

The hearing impaired child is at a disadvantage when it comes to the interactionary and regulatory aspects of speech and language. Group discussions entail complex interactions. It is not acceptable to interrupt. Often the teacher directs who may speak at any given time and invites additional comments. In a more free ranging discussion the individual has to monitor personally what others are saying and formulate any intended contribution. When an appropriate pause ensues this contribution can be introduced. This calls for fairly precise timing. Most adults have had the experience of waiting for an opportunity to arise in order to express their views, only to hear them being propounded by other discussants. Somehow either the chairman's eye has not been caught or others present have managed to exploit the breaks more adroitly. If hearing impaired children are not to be discouraged very early on they need help to have their say.

Hearing impaired children usually have difficulty replying in detail because they have a more limited vocabulary than other children. How much more limited tends to be fairly closely linked to the severity of the hearing loss. Many profoundly hearing impaired children leave school with vocabularies less than average 4 year olds. Those with losses of sufficient magnitude to warrant being on the roll of a partially hearing units frequently barely achieve what might be expected of an 8 year old, as illustrated by examples in the last chapter. Hence there is a paucity of linguistic resources to give detailed answers and explanations. Teachers often ask the class questions in a way that does not give too many clues, so as to check knowledge and understanding most effectively. This sort of approach is almost certain to put the hearing impaired child at a disadvantage. The reader is referred back to the section (p. 54) dealing with the need to provide context.

## Writing: motor and sensory variables

Writing demands the combination of various skills. As has been repeatedly emphasized awareness of sound and limited language development have a very pervasive effect. Even though a degree of competence may be achieved in motor skills it will be subtly different with regard to those aspects which are refined through hearing, especially precise, fine motor movements. Prematurity has been mentioned as a possible cause of hearing impairment. This in itself often leads to varied degrees of motor problems. So some of the skills listed below as being normally acquired by five years of age may still not be well established at secondary level. Individuals with normal hearing will be encountered in secondary schools, who display similar characteristics. Typically they are said to lack motivation. Any written or other forms of recording is not done well and often not completed. Occasionally a better piece of work is produced, i.e. of greater length with fewer crossings out and corrections. This is taken to be an indication that if the requisite amount of effort were always made then this standard could be maintained and improved upon. Such cases as I have assessed frequently exhibit visuo-perceptual motor difficulties. Straight lines cannot be drawn quickly and accurately. When copying seemingly simple geometrical type drawings a variety of distortions, reversals and inversions are often made. The fundamental inability to coordinate hand and eye is thereby revealed. So the reluctance to start upon written work, or do much of an acceptable standard stems from an underlying physical disability, which is the primary cause of the problem. It is not uncommon for those alluded to to have had some minor hearing impairment when younger.

**Table 6: General motor skills**

| Age (years) | |
|---|---|
| 1 | Voluntary release (i.e. makes conscious decision to drop or throw a toy). |
| $1^1/2$ | Transfers an object from one hand to another in order to pick up second object. Builds a tower of bricks (3–4); unwraps small objects. |
| 2 | Can remove outer clothing (i.e. has necessary grip and control). |
| $2^1/2$ | Cuts with scissors (clumsy movements). |
| 3 | Draws a circle; does up buttons. Imitates construction of three cube bridge. |
| $3^1/2$ | Can touch fingers with thumb of same hand sequentially in imitation of a demonstration. Copies a line drawn obliquely. |
| 4 | Draws a cross. |
| 5 | Can copy a star. Uses a dynamic tripod when writing letters. Can translate a two dimensional plan into a three dimensional model using bricks. |

Some motor skills result from normal maturational processes. Head, hand, trunk and leg control cannot be taught in the early stages. Grasping, sitting and walking must wait for changes to occur in the central nervous system. Once a child is able to take steps, the change from flat-footed to heel and toe walking only occurs when myelination of the motor nerves is complete. The ability to move thumb and fingers independently ($3^1/2$ years, see Table 6), is another ability that cannot be taught. In the absence of any abnormality quite high level skills can be taught shortly after the age of $3^1/2$–4 years. In exceptional cases, such as Mozart, very high levels of manual dexterity have been documented. At this age in Japan a technique for training violinists has been perfected. It is certainly not by chance that very rapid, fine hand control is linked to musical ability. The ability to make exceedingly quick, fine auditory discriminations, coupled with a good memory for what is heard, informs the fingers what to do.

Because the capacity for learning fine, motor skills is present in the case of most $3^1/2$–4 year olds, the opportunities must be given to refine them. Usually encouragement is given at home to try and be as self sufficient as possible. This will apply to such things as doing up buttons, tying shoe laces, washing hands, etc. Depending on the home there may be toys to encourage matching, fitting, screwing, and so on. So it is likely the child will arrive at school having practised most common manipulative skills. In the normal course of events we do not need to worry about precisely how skilfully each of these can be performed. We tend to regard them as 'all-or-nothing' skills. As stated earlier this is likely to be a disservice to hearing impaired children. The Interim Report of the Design and Technology Working Group has identified this area as one of importance too: 'pupils will need a knowledge and understanding of the safe use of: hand tools and equipment as diverse as scissors, keyboard, tin opener, whisk, hammer, hacksaw, plane' (p. 35; 2.25.7).

Few activities have no accompanying sound. Tying up shoelaces; undoing a button; drawing a brush lightly across a sheet of sugar paper, even scribbling with a pencil, make their own sounds, though very quiet. For most of the time they will pass unnoticed, except at a subliminal level by those with normal hearing and not at all by the hearing impaired. Always be alert for such sounds. Think what information they are providing. Devise ways to draw a hearing impaired child's attention to them. This will only be possible in quiet surroundings.

Due to the severity of some children's hearing loss it will not always be possible for them to hear the sorts of sounds alluded to, no matter how carefully things are arranged. In such cases attention needs to be drawn to other sensations that are normally disregarded along with accompanying sounds. They are touch, movement and vibration. These are useful in teaching most skilled motor movements especially those related to writing. Activities which draw attention to these sensations are given below.

## Vibrotactile activities

### Sand tray

The sounds associated with sand play have already been mentioned. If the surface is smoothed down patterns may be drawn. Many movements in writing are in an anti-clockwise direction, which appears to be the natural direction for most people to make small, circular movements. Most children imitate circles drawn in this fashion. A small number make a movement in a clockwise direction. This usually calls for direct guidance, that is, holding the child's hand, with index finger extended. (If, due to the child's hearing loss, you are facing him or her – to provide the opportunity for lip reading – remember to reverse all your demonstrations. The same will be true if you are showing vertical lines from top to bottom.) Apart from simple lines and circles other shapes can be drawn, for example spirals and zig-zags. Completely dry sand produces one kind of vibrotactile sensation. When dampened and compacted slightly, greater pressure is needed to make marks. Added to the scraping of the sand against the skin is the feeling of coolness. An advantage of using the sand tray is that quite large movements are made. Gross motor skills are more likely to be reasonably developed than fine finger ones. So no undue stress is involved for making acceptably accurate movements.

## Sandpaper shapes and letters

Froebel and Montessori trained teachers will already be very familiar with these. They were not originally intended for use with hearing impaired children. Their purpose is to make use of the vibrotactile information to reinforce an awareness of the kinaesthetic movements. It is likely they are available in many nursery and infants schools already. If not they can easily be cut from medium grade sandpaper and pasted onto cards. A light wash of colour can be used to make them more attractive in appearance if desired.

## Ribbed plastic letters

Letters can be bought from educational suppliers. If they are traced over with a finger, correct movements flow smoothly over the surface. Going the wrong way leads to resistance, immediately providing feedback that the movements are incorrect.

## Small individual blackboards and chalk

With the refined chalk or pastels now available the vibrotactile element is quite slight. It is still there to a worthwhile degree. The size of the chalk makes it easy to hold and larger movements are made than when writing with a pencil. The shapes used when drawing in sand can be used and refined, in addition to letter practice.

## Kinaesthetic sensation

Kinaesthetic sensations (that is, those associated with making movements) arise when engaged in the activities listed above. The general principle to bear in mind when using them to develop motor skills is to initially exploit gross motor movements. There are now on the market moulded plastic letters onto which a large ball-bearing can be placed. When this is done the ball rolls in the right way to form the letter correctly. First the child is able to watch, then using its finger, trace the same path. The rounded end of a pencil can be used next and finally the letter drawn on a blackboard. At this stage all the movements the child is required to make are rather larger than when writing with a pencil. So bigger muscle groups are involved in a more dynamic way, enhancing the awareness of the kinaesthetic element. Practice with these letters, in the way specified can be followed up with writing on individual blackboards. Accuracy of movements is the primary objective, but speed should not be ignored. Later on very rapid writing movements will be called for, especially if examination courses are taken. Single letters should be made with quick, smoothly flowing movements. This method will also be found of value with children with normal hearing who have hand–eye coordination difficulties, who experience great difficulty in correct letter formation.

I recently used the method with six such children in an ordinary nursery school, referred because they were not responding to the usual teaching approaches. It has to be admitted that the knowledge of phonetics, essential when teaching hearing impaired children who have associated articulation defects, did help with certain aspects of the teaching methods employed. This was particularly true in respect of the vowels. Each child was seen for between five and ten minutes, twice a week. At the end of nine weeks they all knew the names of the letters of the alphabet, the varied sounds made by the vowels, and could write correctly every letter when named. A couple had gone on to joined-up writing. Reading had improved in every case too.

An important feature of the teaching methods employed was the linking of what the children looked at, what they said and what they did. All the stages used in respect of the letter 'a' provide an illustration. The letter was placed in front of the child. Its name was specified. The ball was rolled and the other stages of tracing followed. This still did not guarantee the automatically correct writing on a blackboard. So the ball was placed at the start and the child had to say the name of the letter before pushing the ball. Saying the name then preceded the other activities and succeeded in establishing in advance the correct movements in response to the stimulus of the name. The different ways in which the letter 'a' might be said, that is: front position – as in pat; middle position – as in make; and back position – as in car, were introduced, to avoid too rigid association between the visual form of the letter and its name. Indeed the children were taught to make an appropriate oral response according to whether the vowels were held up in different positions. The equivalence to tongue positions was not pointed out specifically. It is important to always be forward looking and bear in mind future goals, so as to ensure skills relevant to attaining those goals are developed. If this is not done inappropriate habits may be hardened that make change difficult.

One slightly contentious issue involved when teaching is the insistence of standard English. When doing the work described above I did indeed want the children to make the same sounds as I did, since what was being established was the link between the letter and the sound(s). In order to ensure agreement consonance between teacher and taught was essential. Provided they learned and understood the pertinent relationships, how they speak at other times is largely irrelevant.

The stressing of finely controlled movements is important for hearing impaired children as they are likely to bang about, unless explicitly directed to do otherwise. Although emphasis has been placed on skills related to writing, quickness, neatness and quietness should be encouraged with all practical activities. This will apply to: closing doors; lifting chairs so as not to scrape; putting objects down (rulers, jam-jars, etc.). Perhaps the one word that sums up the general goal is gracefulness. The most striking characteristic about any good craftsman is the controlled economy and seeming effortlessness of movements. Some people have a natural aptitude. It is virtually certain hearing impaired children will have to be taught carefully and specifically to reach acceptable levels of competence. This will be especially true with TVEI at secondary level. The handling of tools and drawing aids must be more carefully demonstrated, breaking down what has to be done into component subskills if necessary.

Most of the mechanical aspects of writing have been set out above, emphasising the use of other sensations which are often neglected, namely *vibrotactile, proprioceptive, kinaesthetic,* and *auditory.* In addition to these there are some additional, quite simple mechanical aspects that should be catered for.

## Lighting

If natural lighting is the source then it should come from the left (right for left-handed children). Most artificial lighting tends to be diffuse nowadays, but if it is not then the same will apply as for natural light. If the writing is to be copies then that must be well illuminated too.

## Furniture

Seats should be of such a height that feet may be comfortably flat on the floor, when the knees are bent at a right angle. This makes it easier to maintain the trunk in a good upright position. It will be recalled that the strain of sitting more or less immobile in order to lip read has already been mentioned. So 'sitting comfortably' is of particular importance to hearing impaired children. The table should be of such a height that there is no undue bending or stretching of the elbow. A slightly inclined surface is helpful for writing on. It serves to make what has been written easier to read and also minimizes the changes of arm movement as writing proceeds from left to right. Even highly skilled readers and draughtsmen use sloping surfaces as with lecterns and drawing boards for these reasons.

## Posture

A good upright position should be insisted on at all times. If the child is slumped with weight on the writing arm, instead of the helpful feedback sensations being derived from correct movements, they will be blanked out by the drag. Examples of writing trailing down to the right are usually caused by this. Apart from being unhelpful as far as writing is concerned it does not help with breathing either. If a child has a tendency to droop exercises can be given, e.g. sitting with hands on hips and rotating the trunk or raising hands above the head and stretching gently backwards. The habits formed early in life can be very beneficial later. Back problems are too common anyway, so if what is taught results in nothing more than reducing a liability it will be worthwhile.

## Grip

It is possible to write with the most unorthodox kind of grip, but the dynamic tripod is the most efficient. In the early stages careful attention should be given to developing this. If a child has difficulty, resting the wrist on the edge of the table, then curling the little finger has the result of pulling the fingers into more or less the right position to place the pencil correctly.

If the features listed above are carefully adhered to a good basis will be laid for a well balanced position which will make fluent writing easier to learn. Teachers may be uncertain at what level remediation exercises should be started. The principle to follow is to first identify what developmental stage has been reached. Then, as a rule of thumb it is usually necessary to go back at least one stage to work at the subskills at that level. When the development of *motor skills* was presented earlier, the order listed was in accordance with normal motor development. First, there were large movements that did not call for particularly fine muscle control, such as drawing in sand or on a large blackboard. Once a pencil is used fine coordination is called for. When uneven pressure is a problem, exercises with a stiff bristle brush can draw attention to what needs to be done. First the brush has to be moved over the paper so as not to bend the bristles. Then more pressure can be applied to produce a specified amount of bending. Precisely the same principles of gradation are applied as to breath control. An advantage of using a brush that does not mark is the absence of a visible record of mistakes and flowing movements can be made without fear of error.

## Joining dots and tracing over letters

These activities are commonly used, but unless individually supervised there is no certainty that the correct movements are made and there is nothing about these activities to encourage a free flow. Joining dots can have quite the opposite effect as jerks are made from one to the next. The various other activities suggested do not suffer from these drawbacks.

## *Writing proper*

By the time a child is expected to write words and short sentences there will have been a great deal of pre-writing practice, including in the final stages the writing of individual letters. The reason there has been such an emphasis on perfecting the motor aspects is to make them second nature, executed without any conscious thought. If the instruction is given to write a particular letter the child should be able to do so immediately. Then enquiries about how words are spelled can be written down independently by the child. It was pointed out in Chapter 3 that hearing impaired children's learning tends to be situation specific and they may have difficulty in modifying what has been learned at one stage to accommodate what is learned subsequently and why variations such as those described above are helpful. It was pointed out at the beginning that letters have names and can indicate different sounds when used in words. The once familiar question used when teaching a phonic approach, 'What does that letter say?' is unhelpful. Letters do not *say* anything.

Cursive writing should be encouraged, joining up the letters as soon as the child is expected to write words at all. We think in words not letters. It is the words that must be transformed into written form. So initially anything that has to be written, whether it is what the child wants to say or work to be copied, a check must be made that the child can say it and knows how to spell all the words without having to look. Occasionally a long word which exceeds the child's memory span might be introduced. In that case it is usually possible to break it down into syllables. If the child really cannot remember the word, even when so broken down the exercise is futile.

Why is it necessary to be so pedantic when teaching hearing impaired children to write? Why should they not compile personal dictionaries in the way other children do? Because if they do not hear completely accurately and their own articulation is defective, when they try to say a word they might well mislead themselves by incorrect pronunciation. Examples of this happening abound among children with normal hearing, who write 'fing' and fail to recognize 'thing' in a book. Teachers involved in adult literacy schemes report their pupils often think their reading would improve if they learned to 'talk posh'. They probably would. This is the reason for repeatedly stressing the basics. Unless they are mastered everything else that is superimposed remains unstable and not readily retrievable for practical usage.

# 7  Personality and Emotional Development

It will have become clear by now that hearing impairment not only affects academic progress, it also influences personality development. The 1944 Education Act referred to each child being educated according to age, ability and aptitude. It also led to the categorization of children, which the Warnock Report and the 1981 Education Act aimed to undo. Underlying all three, however, was the need to consider the whole child. Teaching is more than the imparting of information. In some schools the emphasis shifted so strongly towards the consideration of the individual child that there was a danger of staff becoming more like social workers than teachers. The 1988 Act is the pendulum swing back towards an emphasis on facts. But it is not just a reversion to older practices, more the sort of progression referred to by Bruner, with his Spiral Curriculum (Bruner, 1960). Alongside the teaching of facts there must also be a development of skills which enable the children to make use of the facts in innovative ways. This is essential to cope with information technology. Those who have not learned to handle information may suffer from the data deprivation syndrome, now reported in the USA. Individuals feel obliged to look at anything and everything that can be put up on a VDU, for fear of missing anything.

No teacher can be expected to constantly consider the individual personalities and backgrounds of every child in his or her class. None the less, since many hearing impaired children display similar personality characteristic, it is as well to be apprised of certain features. Knowing that certain patterns of behaviour are likely to occur can prevent anxiety or any inclination to self-reproach. Also sensitivity will be enhanced in such a way as to notice warning signals and take steps to defuse any potentially disruptive situation.

Everyone has a personal view of what is meant by *personality, emotions* and *motivation*. Heated arguments are likely to arise if *emotional disturbance* is mentioned. It is not possible to give definitions that will satisfy everyone. The best that can be done is to say how these particular words are used in this context.

## Personality

An individual's personality encompasses all conceivable aspects of their mental life and behaviour. It would be pointless trying to list all the varied facets that have been selected for study at different times. Intelligence, what it is and even whether it exists as an identifiable entity has spawned innumerable publications. The same is true of personality traits such as introversion and extroversion. The psychology of Freud has given rise to fervent adherents and dismissive critics. What remains true is that some people appear to have temperaments that enable them to withstand all sorts of adverse influences whereas others are very vulnerable to stress. Furthermore such traits seem to be present at or even before birth. Hearing impaired children share this characteristic. Some are always cheerful and outgoing, whereas others are sullen and moody. There is the usual range in between the two extremes.

A person's basic temperament is referred to as *endogenous*. Someone who is habitually grumpy attracts the sort of remark, 'Don't bother about her. She's always like it.' A reaction to events is said to be *exogenous*. If one's new car has just been damaged in a crash it is regarded as quite normal for the most cheerful of people to show anger and annoyance. The emotional response is exogenously determined. What follows will indicate that hearing impaired children and adults are subject to many more exogenous factors to upset and annoy them than people with normal hearing.

## Emotions

Emotions are subjective experiences. Some are associated with well-defined physiological changes in the body. Anger and fear are two such. When the individual perceives an annoying or fearful stimulus adrenaline and noradrenaline are released into the blood-stream. Like anything else that gets into the blood-stream it takes time for these hormones to be broken down and a resting state regained. About 20 minutes is a rough guide. When someone is showing signs of either of these emotions we typically try to talk in a soothing way to calm them down. The degree of success and the rapidity depends on the strength of the emotions involved.

Apart from the obvious emotions – fear, anger, love and hate – there are others of a less well-defined nature. Even so these milder emotions – admiration, boredom, concern, distaste, envy and so on are often accompanied by direct physical sensations. Eyes open wide with envy; lips pucker to show distaste. It is an interesting fact that if ever a group of people is asked to list as many emotions as possible the negative ones always predominate. This might be an innate predisposition. Certainly when hearing impaired children are described they are far more frequently described in negative terms than other children.

## Motivation

It is evident that motivation is closely linked with emotions. It is seldom so apparent, except perhaps in very competitive situations. The most extreme example may be witnessed in a boxing match. Even there it is exceptional for an unbridled emotional response to dominate the situation. Everyday motivation is usually a gentler process, leading to productive activities, friendly social interactions and leisure pursuits. There is an inner drive to be engaged.

## Emotional disturbance

We are all subject to a range of emotional responses. It is natural to cry when hurt, either physically or by bereavement. Success produces a joyful response. Shared it can verge on mass hysteria. Wild applause and the throwing of flowers in a concert hall is considered civilized behaviour. Raucous shouts, invading the pitch and throwing beer bottles is a matter for the police to deal with. Most complex societies tolerate a wide spectrum of behaviour. Consequently what is regarded as either normal or deviant varies greatly, both in respect of time and place. If deviant is said to be equivalent to disturbed, then anyone who frequently shows signs of emotional responses that either in terms of frequency or intensity draw undue attention, then that person is likely to be described as emotionally disturbed. What this seems to mean is behaviour which does not seem reasonable to most observers. It does not correspond with the range of cause and effect accepted as normal in a given community.

# Emotional development of hearing impaired children

Emotional and motivational development cannot be considered separately. Pleasant experiences are sought out. What provokes displeasure is avoided. In what way are the experiences of hearing impaired children likely to differ from those of children with normal hearing? Hearing impairment, being an umbrella term, means different categories must be considered separately.

## Severe/profound congenital hearing loss

At birth there has not been much of any auditory experience. The pacifying effect of the mother's steady heart-beat is absent. There is no use in buying a recording to play. The foundations for soothing tones and words to be effective do not exist. So in the event of a tantrum the combined effects of physical restraint and words of comfort are not available. A hearing impaired child will screw up its face and close eyes streaming with tears just like any child with normal hearing. Only touch remains. An angry young child tends to shrug and pull away. As a result the child with a profound congenital loss is likely to experience longer, unremitting outbursts of anger and annoyance, being less open to consolation.

In Western child-rearing practices a baby is often left in a cot. Mother is not usually far away. If the baby cries words of comfort are spoken as a prelude to physical contact. This and the actual sounds of footsteps approaching signal what is about to happen. When the baby cannot hear there is the shock of contact, unheralded by any other signal. When left, as soon as visual contact is broken, there is isolation. The absence of auditory cues subjects the baby to frequent mini-shocks. Reaction to shock is an emotional response accompanied by production of adrenalin. The physiological correlate of angry responses is therefore stimulated repeatedly from an early age.

## Moderate congenital hearing loss

It is probable that the lower frequencies in the speech range can be heard. Also impact noises will be detected. Although auditory experiences are attenuated, in the early stages of development pacifying sounds and crooning will be effective. The tone and not the content is important. Later, when verbal communication is the key element, an inability to understand readily or be able to express thoughts leads to frustration. As might be expected this group of children also display more than usual signs of temper and stubbornness.

## Mild congenital and fluctuating hearing losses

Mild hearing loss can be most provoking. We are all creatures of habit and like everyday life to be predictable. If a child is spoken to and obviously understands in one situation then it is expected he or she will respond in all other situations in which children respond. Yet this is precisely what many children with a mild or fluctuating loss cannot do. For the latter the situation is in some ways worse because on a good day everything is smiles and on a bad (poor hearing) day instructions and explanations are either hard to follow or missed completely. It is about these children that the following comments are most frequently made: 'S/he's ... just being naughty/so moody/lazy/a loner/a day-dreamer/able to hear when s/he wants to/doesn't listen.' The same comments are sometimes made about children with moderate hearing losses and occasionally even those with quite severe ones. They are often an expression of the teacher's frustration. It is not surprising if the attitudes reflected by the comments are conveyed to the child. Since they are hostile attitudes they will provoke angry responses, which might take the form of temper tantrums or withdrawal. Whichever happens to be the case the child's level of motivation will be affected. Why should attempts be made to please someone who is hostile, especially if one is unable to achieve results which are intrinsically satisfying.

## The effect of prolonged stress

Stress makes the person subjected to it more irritable and less efficient. The hearing impaired child is expected to function normally even though deprived of the full range of requisite information. An example of how this can lead to explosions has already been referred to. The boy had gone deaf over a period of months when he was about 8 years old. This was naturally a traumatic experience, but he was resilient and continued to do well in school with the support of a partially hearing unit. His angry outbursts were prompted on each occasion by his teacher continuing to talk while turning to write on the black-board. Already stressed by the efforts he was having to make and then being deprived of lip reading, his only means of following, he went berserk.

## Social isolation

It is a truism to say one can be alone in a crowd. Nearly everyone has had the experience of being the odd one out. The realization of being in such a position then makes it harder to establish contact. Shyness is induced together with anxiety about acceptance. Confident individuals, especially if they make small talk easily, succeed in entering the group. The crucial element is to talk. Most hearing impaired children do not have a ready flow of language. Furthermore if they are to enter into conversation there is a dependence on others to respond clearly. In group situations with a free-for-all element as far as who speaks is concerned, considerable skill is called for. Anyone who does not obey the rules tends to be excluded. Hearing impaired people have to effectively button-hole the one they want to talk to. This is a characteristic of the party bore.

Occasionally I use the make-a-picture story technique. The child is given a variety of pictorial backgrounds (living room; bedroom; classroom; street scene). There are also cut-out figures which can be placed on the pictures to facilitate making up stories. One of the figures is a puppy dog. Hearing impaired children typically people the pictures showing the characters interacting. The dog is placed in a corner and not mentioned. It just sits watching. This is often what happens to them, even with their own families. Parents of hearing impaired children often say that they involve them in everything. This often means little more than taking them along. Think of all the games that are suggested to keep children amused (if not always happy) in the back seats of the car on long journeys. How many of them can be played without relying on hearing to a large extent? Remember that the noise of the car and other traffic makes the wearing of a hearing aid impracticable as the ambient noise masks speech.

Older children who have become hearing impaired to any significant degree may comment on the strain they experience in social situations. They are able to do this because they can compare before and after. If the loss is severe and the quality of their speech has been affected there is the frustration of not being understood in shops. Former friends fade away. Brothers and sisters make some effort, but they have their own friends with whom they can converse readily and share a joke.

Prolonged isolation takes its toll of anybody in its thrall. Behaviour becomes irrational. Paranoia is commonplace. Not surprisingly there is a higher incidence of mental illness among deaf people than in the population at large. Many adults, hearing impaired from childhood, join clubs for others with similar disabilities. There they can find some of the social interaction we all need to maintain our balance.

## Overall personality development

It is dangerous to make generalizations. A few exceptions will always be quoted to suggest they are false. Despite this it may safely be said hearing impaired children tend to be quicker to take offence than other children. Though by no means devoid of a sense of humour, they are less likely to swap jokes and tell humorous anecdotes. Conversely in some situations where it is more considerate to conceal mirth – especially when it involves someone else's misfortune – they might laugh.

There is a tendency to remain self-centred. In order to communicate they often have to focus on one channel and lock onto it. This makes it very difficult to monitor what else is happening at the same time and modulate what is being said or done to take account of the reactions of others.

Mood swings tend to be more frequent and more extreme than average. As mentioned earlier hearing impaired children have been subjected to more events that startle. Language serves not only the purpose of communication. It relates feelings and experiences to each other. This provides a system of checks and balances. Psychotherapy makes use of this fact. Through talk the individual is put in touch with his or her feelings. Language development is always poorer than usual in hearing impaired children and nuances are seldom appreciated. So psychotherapeutic intervention, or the everyday equivalent of talking things through is less effective.

In the course of development internalized value systems grow. There is a central core and associated constellations. This may be explained most easily by thinking of certain political attitudes. A conservationist is likely to approve of organic farming, make a conscious effort to recycle paper and glass, campaign for unleaded petrol and be to the left of any political party supported. Strong views may be held on abortion and alternative medicine. A complex, interlocking set of ideas and beliefs result in fairly predictable reactions. Postal advertising makes greater and greater use of this kind of predictability. People who buy one kind of product are more likely to buy others that fall into a similar (marketing) category. Hearing impaired children tend not to develop such complex personality structures to the same degree as other children. They behave in a more compartmentalized way. As a result there is a greater likelihood of their expressing points of view that conflict when moving from one topic to another, due to the lack of interconnections. It is not possible to rectify this completely, but an integrated teaching approach, highlighting relationships between different aspects, will help.

A further facet of different personality development is a more rigid application of the good/bad, right/wrong type evaluation. It is in effect a way of maintaining a clear cut structure. Faced so often with uncertainty, unambiguous responses are a relief, not calling for further thought. None the less every reasonable opportunity should be taken to come to grips with the grey areas, it may be said paradoxically.

The following two groups of descriptions have been culled from literature about hearing impaired children.

## Group 1

HYPERACTIVE LACK OF CONTROL

The use of the word hyperactive is seldom justified. Hyperactivity is a medical diagnosis and the children so described are almost never still. Hearing impaired children can well appear less settled, as they look around to gain information received clearly by others through hearing. If they wish to talk to someone they will probably have to get close. Whispering across the room is out. Some movement may be accounted for by the need to relax tension built up by holding still to concentrate on lip reading.

IMPULSIVE UNREFLECTION AND UNINHIBITED BEHAVIOUR

This follows from what was said about personality development above. Actions, like moods may be much more self-contained. The experience of others intruding on their thoughts and actions, without warning, makes them unaware that they are behaving any differently when they interrupt: 'Please may I have . . .?/Excuse me please,/Would you mind . . .?' are as often used as a signal of the speaker's intention as a request; the form of words justifying the action. Such subtlety escapes most hearing impaired children, supposing the remarks were heard clearly in the first place. So an angry outburst may ensue as the object in question is seen being taken away. A well-behaved child, by comparison is likely to make a movement or comment to signal the right formula has not been used to consent. If there is any objection a remark such as, 'I'm just going to use it myself,' deters. Group dynamics are modulated in a very sophisticated way in well-controlled situations. Subtlety and sophistication are not characteristics of most hearing impaired children.

ANXIOUS INHIBITION

This arises from uncertainty. It is better to do nothing than make the attempt and get it wrong.

PREOCCUPATION AND OBSESSIVE CONCENTRATION

This applies more to children with severer hearing losses. The lack of a structured auditory environment keeping them apprised of what is going on around has the effect of locking them within their own heads as it were.

AGGRESSIVENESS, ANXIETY AND HOSTILE ISOLATION

Hearing impaired children experience much higher levels of isolation and resultant frustration than other children. What cannot be expressed in words is more likely to be expressed in violence. Uncertainty leads to anxiety. Others are observed conforming. The hearing impaired child makes mistakes and is corrected. What has probably not been noticed are the times when other children have been corrected. So he or she may finish up with the erroneous impression of being the only one corrected and feel less able. A natural reaction is to withdraw from situations where it is not possible to compete on an equal footing. 'Why don't you join in?' Through not knowing how, would be the answer if only the reason were known and capable of being expressed. Not being part of the group is often perceived as rejection. Rejection is then equated with hostility – QED, the hearing impaired child shows signs of hostile isolation.

## Group 2

LACK OF PERSISTENCE

In Chapter 4 various forms of auditory feedback from everyday occupations were described. They can serve the function of indicating what is about to happen and when the expected event has taken place. The change of tone as a piece of wood is nearly sawn through and the final note as the last cut is made has the effect of satisfyingly rounding off the whole. It is like the final chord of a piece of music. These and many other experiences help to show we are on the right track and underpin motivation. Hearing impaired children want feedback too. Often they will give up if it is delayed, not having developed the normal degree of motivation which is so greatly stimulated by verbal means. By giving up the goal will not be reached. Necessary experience and practice to proceed to the next stage is thereby missed, largely due to lack of comprehensive auditory input.

INABILITY TO APPLY WHAT HAS BEEN LEARNED IN LIFE SITUATIONS

This comment refers to the practical part of lessons, intended to reinforce explanations, prior to recording. Unless great care is taken to make the activity crystal clear together with the requisite language it is probable the hearing impaired child will imitate the motions of the other children, but fail to make the relevant observations about the operations being performed personally. Imitative behaviour of this kind may produce an end product that looks much the same as the others, but for the child all that has happened has been a number of disjointed movements, lacking coherence. Furthermore it is virtually certain the activities will not have been accompanied by internal, verbal rehearsal, e.g.

First draw the shape(s); cut round; bend the flaps; apply the glue – taking care not to go over the edge or it will spoil the finish; put the paste where it can't be knocked over; press together firmly; wipe off any extra; place the model on the side to dry.

The anxiety aroused from looking at what others are doing will also interfere with noticing all kinds of little details. As curves and corners are negotiated with the scissors, unless correct anticipatory movements are made, errors will arise. The optimal amount of glue on the brush has to be gauged. The positioning of the pieces must be judged precisely. Often the teacher will give hints about these matters when going round to see how the children are getting on. They will alert the child being addressed and also the others who overhear. Once more the hearing impaired child is likely to be the loser. Such detail has to be specified in the initial instructions. Careful planning is imperative at all times.

INABILITY TO TRANSFORM OLD LEARNING TO NEW

This relates to the compartmentalization already mentioned earlier. The inflexibility of certain personality structures makes accommodation of new information or transformations more difficult. Something considered right before now has to be accepted as wrong. The reader is probably experiencing some exasperation at the simplistic dichotomy. That is what has to be explained to the hearing impaired child. Partial changes do not invalidate the whole.

POOR STUDY HABITS

The reasons hardly need any further explanation. Many subskills have to be called into play for study to be effective. They have to be martialled and applied consistently. These are all linked by a network of language and depend upon both knowledge and personality variables.

## *Tendency to have the learning of one skill interfering with what has been previously learnt*

It is normal to remember best what has occurred most recently. If the facts learned tie in with what has been learned well previously, there is mutual reinforcement. Recent learning is facilitated and past learning made more readily accessible. This is what happens after prolonged study and accounts for the very large body of knowledge specialists in any field can draw upon at will. Recall of information (and skills) seems to depend on tags. If an appropriate tag can be grasped retrieval is fairly simple. Something on the tip of the tongue may first be identified by a rhythm or a sound. Then the sought for facts are summoned up.

At a time when children are crystallizing and structuring their sensory impressions by attaching labels, hearing impaired children are not able to learn words so easily. The tags are missing. Instead of clarifying previous learning, new information and skills make it more amorphous and less easily accessed. It is for this reason the need for careful reinforcement of new concepts and the associated vocabulary has been repeatedly stressed.

## Implications for the classroom

It is not going to be possible to overcome all of the effects of hearing impairment on emotional and behavioural development. A great deal of sensitivity and patience is required to minimize them. Precisely what is happening should be analysed in order to decide how best to intervene and develop social skills. Social skills in this context are simply those forms of behaviour which make an individual an acceptable member of the community. As is well known, the process of socialization starts at birth. The fact the baby is totally dependent on the mother means she is able to shape behaviour. Animal experiments have shown how the feeding can be used to reinforce desired behaviour patterns. To some extent the same is true with human beings. With people the situation is very much more complex, especially once language can be used to communicate with others and equally importantly with oneself. Hearing impaired children often need a lot of encouragement. So although it is gratifying to be given rewards the focus should be on enjoyment of the activity. If it is properly understood and within the child's competence, even simple practice can give pleasure. It may seem somewhat precious to make remarks such as, 'Wasn't it nice to do that so neatly/quickly/to work so hard', etc. But they do serve to link enthusiasm for the activity not simply the end product or an anticipated reward. Also if more praise and tangible rewards are given to a hearing impaired child they will be debased in value, apart from affecting the attitudes of other children.

### Practical steps

1     The teacher is usually the focal point of the classroom. Ensure the hearing impaired child is always in the best position to see and hear.

2     There are other times when the contributions from the class are of prime importance. Unless steps are taken to integrate the hearing impaired child in all the activities then he or she will effectively become one of two classes being taught simultaneously.

3    Choose two or three children in the class with whom the hearing impaired child can be paired for certain activities? It is better to have two or three rather than just one who might be overburdened with responsibility. Also different styles of working will be illustrated, apart from exposing the hearing impaired child to a wider variety of language – since each individual has idiosyncrasies.

4    Encourage the changing of roles occasionally. The hearing impaired child can be primed to pass information to the partner, so as not to be always in a subservient position.

5    Use stories, role play and incidents that occur in the daily life of the school to illustrate the ways in which people show consideration and avoid upsetting each other.

6    Whenever it is necessary to correct or criticize try to temper remarks by alluding to some positive feature that can be identified. This can sometimes be achieved by framing the comments in the form of a question, e.g. 'Can we look to see if this is right?/Are you sure you spell it that way?/Are you ready now?/Did you say sorry when you bumped . . .?' etc.

Very often a confrontational situation can be avoided in this way. The child is required to make an active response instead of being stopped in its tracks. One thing is certain. It is never possible to always do the right thing and some sulks and/or tantrums are bound to occur with young hearing impaired children. How older ones respond will depend on temperament and the nature of their personalities. A firm, gentle approach is likely to be the most effective. If it is ever necessary to actually hold a child do not grip so as to either dig your fingers or completely encircle the child's wrist or arm. This produces a reflex action to get free. The palms of the hand against the upper arms is supportive. Holding over the top of the shoulder is felt as threatening. Always bear in mind the most basic types of reaction and how to deal with them. Also with hearing impaired children it may in times of stress be necessary to think of how you would deal with younger children, as emotional development tends to be delayed along with language.

Be aware of your body language. The shaking of a fist to denote anger is obvious, as is a driver scratching the top of his head when he feels guilty about cutting up another motorist. Most of the time we send out less evident signals. Leaning towards or over is perceived as threatening. Drawing back indicates avoidance and dislike. A brow furrowed in concentration (e.g. to discern imperfect speech) can look very much like a frown. Groups of adolescents sometimes nod towards and grin at others, to make them feel paranoid about being laughed at. Other children then ask, 'Had your pennyworth them?' when noticing they are being looked at. Hearing impaired children are more sensitive than usual to body language, especially if it appears to be conveying a negative message and are much more likely to misread it. A joke shared with one child and the smile alighting on another, is easily construed if the joke has not been heard, as being laughed at. Children with normal hearing complain about others looking at them as indicated. The same is true for hearing impaired children, usually in a more extreme form. This was exemplified in a residential setting. The sign for 'bad' is to clench the fist and raise the little finger. One girl persistently burst into tears and complained bitterly about the girl opposite at tea times. There appeared to be no justification for this. Then it was noticed that the girl complained of cocked her little finger when lifting her tea-cup. The look in her eyes indicated she did indeed intend to sign, 'You are bad,' to the one opposite. This is cited to show how observant the teacher needs to be of signs, gestures and movements, since these are likely to activate the more primitive responses which are latent in all of us. With hearing impaired children, the thin veneer of civilization, largely patinated through the medium of language, is likely to be flawed due to their less sophisticated language development.

Although hearing impaired children may at times appear to have clusters of negative traits, they are as likeable and affectionate as any other child, but more tender loving care may be needed to make this apparent. Given consistent support and encouragement a more equable temperament may be established, alongside consistent application and stable work habits. Even children with profound hearing losses can then take their place alongside their normally hearing peers. Two recent school leavers come to mind as exemplars. One joined an international architects' practice. The other in the first six months of his apprenticeship made such a good impression that he has been guaranteed work as a stone mason, restoring cathedrals, for the rest of his life, if he so wishes.

# 8 Careers

## Background

Early educational establishments for the deaf, in common with orphanages and the poor house, gave their children vocational training. These were commonly carpentry, shoe repairing and other manual trades for the boys; needlework, laundering and housekeeping skills for the girls. Those destined to live in the country would be expected to become farm labourers, alongside many of their kinsfolk. As a greater variety of opportunities became available for the population at large, the range of possible occupations for the hearing impaired expanded accordingly. There remain a number of jobs which are not suitable for anyone with severe hearing impairment.

An example of an unexpected difficulty arose when a profoundly hearing-impaired girl left school. She wanted to be a hairdresser. Her speech was unintelligible except to those familiar with the deaf. Her ability to lip read was insufficient to follow everyday conversation. Although she might have been able to learn to manage the mechanical aspects of hairdressing, instructions from the clients and conversations with them would have been out of the question. By chance a member of staff had a brother who had recently started a wig-making factory. Their parents were both deaf, so a sympathetic attitude already existed.

Arrangements were made for the girl to go and work in the factory, training being given on the job. She lasted just a fortnight. The wigs were expensive, human hair being tied one strand at a time onto the base. What the girl could not do was make the finely controlled movement to make the hairs tight without snapping them. For no good reason everyone with normal hearing seems to know what a hair feels like just before it snaps with a ping. This helps in judging the precise tautness required in wig-making.

Another school-leaver who had gone to Mary Hare Grammar School went into accountancy. Again family connections had helped. He felt he had not been given the opportunities his abilities merited. Most of what he did was straightforward hack work. The problem was his inability to use the telephone. Many clients want to be able to call their accountant and discuss their affairs.

## Current careers options

Most trades are open to hearing impaired people, though in times of high unemployment and a high level of competition for jobs, they will be at a disadvantage. Two examples cited at the end of the last chapter show what is possible, though it must be pointed out both have very equable personalities and were of above average ability. In service industries most openings will be the poorly paid ones, where there is minimal contact with the public at large.

This will be particularly true for those with severe hearing losses, whose speech is not clear and who have to lip read.

The Doncaster College for the Deaf runs residential courses for deaf and partially hearing students, in order to overcome this problem as far as possible. The courses range from foundation courses in Art and Design through Business Studies to Electronic Engineering and Computing Technology. For the more practically inclined there are Brickwork and allied technology courses as well as catering and hairdressing. Students gain qualifications such as City and Guilds, HND (BTec Higher National Diplomas), where the theoretical content is as important as the practical. The Centre For the Deaf, part of the City Literary Institute in London aims to provide similar opportunities for training on a day basis. To benefit from courses with a high level of theoretical input the students have to be of above average ability and have well-developed language skills. This is of course equally true for individuals with normal hearing.

The careers options are now wider than at any time in the past, thanks to the computer screen and telephone links. The Royal National Institute for the Deaf have a facility whereby subscribers can call in. The hearing impaired caller types in the message, which the operator relays orally to the receiver. He or she responds orally and this is typed back to the hearing impaired person's screen terminal. This sort of link has removed one of the obstacles during normal working hours. Naturally this facility is of most importance to those engaged in professional activities. But they and those employed in manual occupations, which will include catering, hairdressing and draughting, as well as the more obvious ones of bricklaying, plumbing and car maintenance, suffer from a disadvantage. While they are looking at what they are doing they cannot be talking, or at least listening to what others are saying. This makes the work-place much more isolated for them. This may be illustrated by someone working as a plasterer. While putting the plaster on with the float and levelling off, a proficient and experienced plasterer can carry on a discussion with his mate, about a football team or any other subject of interest. Also a new batch of plaster can be called for or instructions given to start cleaning up. A person with a hearing loss of such magnitude as to need to lip read is denied this type of social intercourse while directly engaged in his craft. It is the experience of this type of isolation that has led some hearing impaired people to start work enthusiastically and then discover there is something missing. That something is constantly being in touch with others. It is a feature that helps to make routine and perhaps intrinsically boring work acceptable on a long-term basis.

Hearing impaired people can now enter most professions. Notable exceptions are medicine; the law and performing arts in which the musical accompaniment is an essential feature. In the case of medicine there are commonplace diagnostic techniques which depend on hearing. Some investigative procedures are of necessity conducted in positions which preclude the possibility of the physician lip reading anything the patient says. At least one person has overcome all the obstacles and successfully completed her training as a dentist. In the chair none of us has much opportunity for saying anything intelligible anyway.

The legal profession is perhaps one of the most dependent on linguistic competence. In each branch there is a very extensive technical vocabulary, used to convey concepts most people in the street are totally unaware of. An idea of the complexities are readily obtained by reading in the newspapers any Law Report of a judgement given in the Court of Appeal. The effect hearing impairment has on language development means that even if in a very exceptional case an individual were able to understand the written accounts, actual participation in a court situation could not be sustained. Hearings often last for days and can go on for months. The necessary arrangements to ensure a hearing impaired person could follow everything that was said at all times just would not be feasible. It is for the same reason that on the rare occasions hearing impaired people appear in court, especially those who have to rely on an interpreter can be at a disadvantage.

The performing arts appear an unlikely destination for hearing impaired children. In the field of classical music it is necessary to have normal, or in many cases better than normal hearing, especially for ensemble playing. The most pianissimo of sounds can be a cue for the other players. The critical importance of acute hearing for the development of manual dexterity ensures no hearing impaired person ever acquires the technical skills to be a solo player, to say nothing of the musicianship entailed. Readers might have seen on television a xylophone player, reported to be deaf after giving her performance. Her speech was virtually normal, so it is probable that her hearing loss is acquired. Also the use of the word 'deaf' does not give any real indication of any useful residual hearing. When she was asked how she kept in time with the accompaniment her answer was very forthright. She said that she did not. The accompanyist had to follow her. In effect she was playing alone.

Ballet is precluded for the same reasons as those already given. Some hearing impaired people have despite all the difficulties entered the acting profession. They are exceptional. On a different plane a theatre for the deaf has been created. In the main the performances are for the hearing impaired community. Carl Campbell, a very talented dancer and teacher is now training deaf adolescents modern dance to a remarkably high standard. Even so it is unlikely they could expect to perform professionally, other than in a specialized setting.

Hearing impaired teachers and hearing impaired social workers now exist, typically to work with hearing impaired children. The sort of pitfall that can occur was witnessed when a profoundly hearing impaired teacher was taking a class of similarly affected children. One boy looked up and said, 'Aeroplane,' when one passed overhead. The teacher's response was to scold him and say that they were not talking about aeroplanes, not having heard it. Apart from congenitally hearing impaired staff in these fields there are the large numbers in these and other professions who have some degree of presbycusis, the high frequency hearing loss that affects everyone to varying degrees as they get older. Older practitioners who have become hard of hearing can continue in certain fields, usually those concerned with community health, where they are mainly performing a screening function.

I had a routine check at work and the doctor concerned, noticing my involvement with hearing impaired children, asked my advice about hearing aids. At the time he was taking my blood pressure and I was curious to know how he detected the point at which the pressure was read. Normally a stethoscope is used. He confessed that while he actually held one against the patients' arms he just waited to see when the mercury in the manometer moved. Since I had come across another doctor in a similar position I was able to advise him about stethoscopes with built-in amplification. This account illustrates once more the difference between acuity and function. Having acquired his skills when he had normal acuity, the doctor was able to function effectively by making use of alternative strategies. For the initial acquisition of skills normal acuity had been crucial.

When caring for patients there are many situations which call for a good ability to hear. Electronic monitoring devices make audible signals to sound an alert. Stentorian breathing may be a sign of distress. Whimpering calls for attention. Hearing aids deprive the wearer of a clear sense of the direction of the source of sound, supposing it were detected in the first place amid all the ambient noise. So not recruiting hearing impaired people into the medical and paramedical professions is not discriminatory.

For most hearing impaired children their work prospects are likely to be in the skilled and semi-skilled areas. Opportunities vary from region to region. Some are fortunate in getting opportunities with a sympathetic employer, who may – as with cases cited above – have a particular reason for taking hearing impaired school-leavers. Most go on to some form of further education, after the age of 16. The emphasis is often on the improvement of communication skills and further development of the maturing process. What career any individual might pursue is of course dependent on many variables. In some areas there are specialist careers officers who can give advice and guidance. There are also organizations which can at times be of assistance too. A list of useful addresses is given at the end of the book. This was made available by the Royal National Institute for the Deaf, a voluntary organization that is always ready to give assistance and advice on every aspect of hearing impairment. They also have a library which is open to the public for both research and lending purposes. From personal experience I can say that the staff there have been the most knowledgeable and helpful it has been my pleasure to come across.

It will have been clear from the chapter on emotions that the hearing impaired often display characteristics regarded as immature and some always retain a degree of naivety. Only by teaching hearing impaired children as effectively as possible, at every stage of their school career can they be given the opportunity of being effectively prepared for the widest range of work situations. It is hoped that this book may have given some pointers as to how this might be achieved.

# 9   Historical Perspectives

In Chapter 2 it was pointed out that a genetically determined hearing loss does not usually affect the general health or intellectual potential of the child, whereas other causes, for example rubella and extreme prematurity, can result in global damage. At one time many of the children in the latter categories would not have survived infancy. This is mentioned because when the historical development of 'deaf education' is considered, those who were taught were predominantly physically healthy children whose hearing loss was caused by a recessive gene. A small proportion had lost their hearing as a result of infections, which could have occurred before or after the acquisition of speech and language.

## Early educational provision for the deaf

There are records of deaf people having been educated in Roman times, but it was only from the sixteenth century on that provision became widespread. Ponce de Leon (1520–84) is usually credited with being the first person to teach a deaf person to speak. It took a great deal of time and patience. He was helped by only having one royal pupil. The experience he gained and the methods he devised were taught to others. Education was largely in the hands of the clergy. Therefore it is not surprising they were taught to finger spell. Finger spelling had been devised by monks in silent orders, to communicate without breaking their vows of silence.

Bonet published a book in 1620 on finger spelling for use in teaching deaf people. In 1789, the Abbé De l'Epée wrote *The True Manner of Instructing the Deaf and Dumb, Confirmed by Long Experience*. Systems of signs had evolved among deaf communities so not every letter had to be individually indicated as with finger spelling. This was a piecemeal process and signs peculiar to individual institutions and locations arose. An example of how localized a sign could be was the picking between the teeth with a thumbnail denoting 'Monday'. The school where it arose always served rice pudding on Monday. De l'Epée familiarized himself with the sign system being used by one particular group of deaf individuals and formalized it for his publication.

Finger spelling follows normal orthographic rules, being directly equivalent, letter for letter, to writing. The signs and sign systems which evolved among hearing impaired communities moved further and further away from the strict correspondence to the written form. In their more developed forms they could only be understood by the initiated. Furthermore correct grammatical syntax was not followed. It was the deviation from the norm which led to later condemnation of manual signs as a means of communication in this country. It may be postulated that the deviation resulted from De l'Epée's teaching as he naturally used French grammar. British Sign Language has strong affinities with Latin grammar.

## The emergence of the oral tradition in Britain

In England the possibility for educating the deaf was publicised as a result of Dr William Holden (1616–98) teaching the 22 year-old Whalley to speak, using the manual alphabet for support. His pupil transferred to the care of Dr John Wallis at the age of 25. A year later the young man was paraded around giving readings from the Bible. Wallis published the details of 'his' method in the Royal Society's Journal, much to the fury of Dr Holden. On the strength of his famous success Dr Wallis was entrusted with another deaf pupil. Unlike Whalley who did not go deaf until the age of five, the other man was prelingually deaf. His progress is shrouded in obscurity.

Thomas Braidwood worked in Scotland. He made a name for himself in 1715. His first much publicised deaf pupil had normal hearing up to the age of three. On the strength of this initial success he set up a school in Edinburgh, taking deaf children from rich families. He did attempt to raise funds so he could take in others but failed and was considerably embittered. Francis Green in 1873 wrote, on the basis of his observations at Braidwood's school,

> The education of deaf children must be the work of time and unremitted perseverance, for years under the constant eye of the teacher who gives 'line upon line and precept upon precept, here a little and there a little', not only in school but at meals, in walking, playing, etc. And upon all occasions making a lesson out of every suitable occurrence (cited by Edward L. Scouten).

Samuel Heinicke (1727–90) wrote a book in which he gave various Principles of Instruction. Just three (his numbering) will give the flavour.

1    The knowledge of a thing precedes its naming. The education of the deaf must therefore proceed from intuitive instructions.

2    Learning speech, which depends on hearing is only possible by substituting another sense for hearing and this can be no other than taste. (As it happened he chose substances that naturally make one curl up one's tongue, like vinegar for 'ee' and wormwood for 'eh'. Water was also used. Being bland it signified a relaxed, open 'ah', which must have been a relief.)

8    As soon as they have learned to speak they should converse with one another, or the hearing and *not use signs*.

Heinicke incidentally has been thought of as the first pure oralist. The oral tradition was established in this country by the Dutchman, William Van

Praagh. He was paid to come in 1867 by the Baroness Rothschild to teach Jewish deaf children in Whitechapel. Through his efforts the Association for Oral Instruction of the Deaf and Dumb was formed in 1871. As well as being the headmaster of the school for children he also started a training course for teachers. Van Praagh was succeeded by Schontheil. In Germany Schonteil had been accustomed to highly qualified teachers who had undergone lengthy training, not the somewhat cursory in-house courses run by Van Praagh. He persuaded the Royal Commission on the Blind and Deaf to set up much more rigorous training course. To this day teachers of the blind and teachers of the deaf are the only ones who have to have a specialist qualification. A then important part of such courses was training in phonetics and learning about articulatory movements. This was necessary as teachers had to actually teach the children to speak, as well as the more formal parts of the curriculum. In a sense teachers of the deaf preceded Speech Therapists in their dealings with speech pathology, though only in relation to that arising from hearing defects.

A wide variety of techniques were developed to stimulate, encourage and refine the speech of congenitally hearing compared individuals. Deaf babies often start to babble normally, but because they cannot hear either other peoples' voices or their own, they stop vocalizing. Later when education starts they have to be specifically taught how to make their vocal cords vibrate, how to shape their lips and tongue and control their breath. For people with normal hearing such abilities develop without any conscious effort. Because hearing impaired people have to exert conscious control, their efforts are never as fluent or readily understood as natural speech.

## The establishment of the oral method

By 1880 there was enough interest in the education of the deaf to hold the International Congress on the Deaf and Dumb in Milan. It decided in favour of the oral method of instruction. A conference of Heads of Institutions for the Deaf and Dumb was held in this country in 1887. They visited the Jewish Deaf School 'to observe the effects of good oral teaching'. As hearing loss was their only handicap many of the pupils succeeded. It should be remembered there were none of the distractions that beset children nowadays. Also the curriculum was much more circumscribed. Older children were given trade training: shoe-repairing and carpentry for the boys; laundering, cookery and needlework for the girls.

With the advent of compulsory education, residential schools with a wide catchment area continued. Day schools were also opened in large cities, following the example once more of the Jewish school. At that time families, especially Jewish families were much more closely knit. But day provision is very different from boarding. Other members of the child's family often do not have the time, ability or inclination to communicate – other than in a most rudimentary way. So instead of being in the company of others as they were in

Braidwood's school, who are equally willing to 'talk' and provide opportunities for learning, the wakeful hours out of school frequently do not provide an opportunity to learn more language. Children with normal hearing learn a lot incidentally from other peoples' conversation. The same is true of hearing impaired children, only they do it through looking. But they have to be in an environment where the communication is in such a form they can learn incidentally. This comment remains as true today as it ever has for children born into families where everyone else has normal hearing.

The Jewish school had a change of heart and became residential when Lord Stern gave his house in south London to it. It was still dedicated to the oral method. There was flexibility, however. Children's need to relax was recognized and the use of signing was permitted in the course of social contact outside the classroom. It was oral in the way that would have been understood by Samuel Heinicke in the eighteenth century.

The pupils who attended the Residential School for Jewish Deaf Children (where the author taught for a number of years) were bound together by their hearing difficulties and their religion. Not surprisingly they formed a club which still flourishes. Quite naturally the club was and is a place where individuals are likely to meet spouses. Communication there is largely through speech (albeit not always easily understood by those who are not familiar with the speech of the deaf). This speech is nearly always accompanied by signing. This is important in social situations. When there is total dependence on lip reading speakers have to be face to face if communication is solely through speech. Sufficient is picked up by others to the side, if signs are used to clarify what is being said. Try looking in a mirror and without using your voice say 'peas' then 'beans'. See how much difference you can see. If you do this you will appreciate how any sign to help make the necessary distinction assists understanding enormously.

## Higher educational provision for the deaf

The Mary Hare Grammar school was set up to provide an academic education for deaf children. The Residential School for Jewish Deaf Children had many successful candidates. This was in spite of the fact many were profoundly hearing impaired from birth. The reason for their success was often because they had deaf parents who taught them to communicate long before they received any formal education. In this respect the deaf parents behaved like any others. The difference between the deaf parents and normally hearing parents who have a hearing impaired child is the deaf ones know how to communicate with the hearing impaired. They structure the hearing impaired child's behaviour and responses so as to notice communication directed at them as soon as the child can make any independent movement.

Colleges of Further Education have also set up courses for the hearing impaired, in addition to providing support teaching for students following main-

Colleges of Further Education have also set up courses for the hearing impaired, in addition to providing support teaching for students following mainstream courses. At one time they were also able to extend this support into work situations, but this has all stopped as a result of the cut-backs.

## Old controversies resurface

A last ditch attempt to stamp out manual methods of communication was made by the Ewings, who ran the Teacher Training Course for Teachers of the Deaf in Manchester. The use of signing to communicate was anathema. Parents were advised to sit on their hands rather than use any gesture to help their hearing impaired child understand. A film called *Mandy*, made in the 1950s, publicised the work of the Manchester school. I trained there and vividly remember my first day as a qualified Teacher of the Deaf on Residential duty. In the evening I was in sole charge of children ranging from 3 to 16 years old. That night I had a nightmare. I emerged from an underground station in a strange city. Every attempt to ask directions was met by glazed looks. All the people looked blankly before gliding away. They were obviously all drug addicts. On waking the explanation was obvious. My training had left me totally unable to communicate effectively with deaf children.

The Ewings were very influential in forming the policies that governed the educational approach used in schools in this country. The National College for Teachers of the Deaf, espoused their cause in support of the 'Oral Method'. Since the College was able to set examinations and award the qualification needed by Teachers of the Deaf, anyone opting for the in-service method of training was guaranteed to be an adherent of the oral method.

A final boost to the oral method was given by the development of various aids to hearing. Adults who had become hard of hearing were helped by ear-trumpets and then cumbersome, battery operated aids. Some 'hearing impaired' children could also be helped in a similar way. The ones who responded best were those who had moderately severe hearing losses. For them unamplified speech was just a mumble. Speech when amplified was heard almost normally. As so often happens a particular approach is hailed as a panacea. It was only necessary to improve hearing aids and all 'hearing impaired' children could be taught like ordinary children. This mistaken belief led to some training courses dropping specific training on how to teach deaf children to speak. As Donald F. Moores observed, 'Ironically, improvements in methods of teaching speech seemed to come to an end at the same time the oral-only philosophy became dominant.'

It is now everyday practice to issue large numbers of expensive and sophisticated electronic aids to children with profound hearing losses, without any careful differential diagnosis. Unfortunately their use does not necessarily lead to better linguistic achievements or clarity of speech for the children involved. The issuing of aids to all and sundry is a defensive reaction. Nobody can criticize if the aids are issued because it has become standard practice. If hearing aids are not issued critics can allege that all that might be done has not been done. So ENT Consultants make a reflex response and write the necessary prescription.

There are still deaf people alive today who were taught before hearing aids were given to children. In some cases their command of language and the quality of their speech is superior to those taught subsequently with the aid of the most up-to-date technology. These remarks are not intended to denigrate the use of all hearing aids. Because of their enormous value to some hearing impaired children it made sense for the Inner London Education Authority to open the first Partially Hearing Unit in 1958. More have been opened since and widely copied elsewhere.

The children who go to partially hearing units usually have sufficient hearing to learn a certain amount of speech and language naturally, by wearing hearing aids. In the main they learn much more quickly than profoundly hearing impaired children and their scholastic attainments tend to come halfway between those of children with profound losses and children with normal hearing. Degree of hearing loss is not the only determinant, innate potential is obviously of great importance. When other factors are taken into consideration there tends to be a fairly direct relationship between degree of hearing loss and attainments. This includes quality of speech.

Medical techniques now succeed in keeping children alive who might otherwise have died. Antibiotics frequently save children with meningitis from dying. But the drugs themselves can damage the auditory nerves and the disease itself often results in some degree of brain damage. The population in schools for the hearing impaired has changed. Not only children of normal intellectual potential and healthy physiques attend. Children with varying degrees of learning difficulty are among their number. Since the inception of the oral tradition of educating the hearing impaired, an increasing number of 'oral failures' have appeared on the scene. The unlucky failures are eased through the system. Those slightly more fortunate are transferred to the ultimate horror – schools where signing is still used, but only after a lot of valuable educational time has been wasted.

## Deaf people find their voice

The wheel has come nearly full circle. It has been encouraged in part by Speech Therapists who use Makaton, a variant of British Signing, to teach children and adults with severe learning difficulties. In most schools for the hearing impaired a combined method is used. Children are taught and encouraged to speak and lip read. Their understanding of the spoken word is assisted by signs which are easily understood. Everyone naturally uses some signs, as when beckoning a child to approach or holding up one's hand, to indicate 'stop'. In an educational setting the manual signs are developed to be the equivalent of 'signed, exact English'. Every spoken word can be accompanied by a sign or if one does not exist, finger spelling. Children who previously failed the system, by not learning through the 'oral method' are now encouraged to communicate. Once concept development is facilitated there is the motivation to speak. Unless an individual has coherent thoughts and something to say, speech remains an unnecessary frippery. To repeat Samuel Heinicke's first principle, 'the education of the deaf must therefore proceed from intuitive instruction'.

Sign language is now recognized as a language in its own right. Professor Stokoe has argued (lecture given on 13.12.77 at UCL) that some misconceptions have arisen because normally hearing observers failed to notice the fine detail contained in sign language. Filmed recordings were made and then slowed down. Syntactic elements thought to be absent in sign language became apparent. When making an analysis of sign language it is necessary to simultaneously take account of three features: the active part(s) of the body, e.g. the hand; the action(s) i.e. the nature of the movement and its direction; the location – where the movements are made and their relationship to the face and other parts of the body. Sipola (cited by Professor Stokoe, see bibliography) has revealed that the mode of movement is also important. A noun as opposed to a verb can be indicated by either a smooth movement or a jerky one. If you make a wiping motion with your hand that could be an instruction to clean. A quicker, slightly truncated movement could mean the object is clean.

The acceptance of sign language (and its being made visible on television screens), means hearing impaired people are no longer treated so much as second class citizens. They are making their voices heard, no longer content to be told by experts what is best for them.

# Appendix I
# Aide Memoire for Language Acquisition, Reading and Writing Skills

This *aide memoire* is intended for reference purposes, so that in the event of a teacher having a hearing impaired child in a mainstream class, salient points can be checked. The greatest attention has naturally been given to language development. Only major areas are covered. For more detailed analysis reference would have to be made to a book like *Grammatical Analysis of Language Disability* (Crystal, Fletcher and Garman, 1976). Ideally the format should enable the user to look across at the varied levels of attainments in the areas alluded to. Unfortunately this is not possible in the present context and therefore it has to be presented sequentially.

## Classroom Organization

Is the hearing impaired child positioned so as to have the most opportunities for lip reading when necessary:

- you
- other children?

- Is lighting appropriately sited and adequate? Ensure the child is not faced by glare.
- Is a board (or overhead projector) readily available on which to write key words and phrases?
- Are record keeping facilities available to monitor any language/speech difficulties?
- Are arrangements in place for easy daily checking and local maintenance of aid(s)? (Spare batteries, leads, charger for radio-aid.)

## Articulation and general speech production

### Breath control

- Does the child have frequent colds?
- Is a good posture normally maintained?
- Is the child as active as the others (a) in the playground (b) in PE?
- Can a steady airstream be: maintained; modulated?

## Voice quality

- Does the child speak at normal loudness?
- Is speech: breathy; of normal resonance and timbre; harsh or creaky?

## Articulation

- Normal vowel sounds. (Note any that are unusual. Are there any rhymes, songs or poems which would give practice in them?)
- High frequency consonants (s, k, t, f, p, sh, ch, z).

## Intonation and pitch

- Is the general tone of voice flat?
- Can the child sing in tune?

# Listening skills

- Understands by listening alone: up to 3ft; more than 3ft; outdoors; unaided; with aid.
- *Lip reading*: usually unnecessary; definitely helpful; essential.
- *Attention span for stories*: short; variable; average; good?
- *Memory* (for discrete facts): poor; variable; average; good?
- *Auditory discrimination* (source; distance; direction; pitch) of:everyday sounds; musical sounds.
- Identification of well-known characters (pop-singers; TV personalities, etc.).

# Language and conversational skills

## Vocabulary

- *Pronouns*: I; me; you; he; him; she; her; it; we; us; they; them; me; my; mine; your; yours; his; hers; its; ours; theirs; -self; -selves.
- *Prepositions*: in; on; under; near; by, etc.
- *Adjectives*: knows comparative and superlative forms.
- *Adverbs of time, place and manner*: soon; later; far; close; quickly; quietly, etc.
- *Verbs*: present (am -ing); future (will); past (-ed and irregular forms); subjunctive (would).

## *Sentence structure*

- *Age appropriate*: immature; telegraphic; monosyllabic.
- *Complex sentences used including*: phrases; clauses; recursions.

## *Questions*

- *Questions are asked*: frequently; infrequently; never.
- *Uses*: who; what; where; when; how; why.
- *Answers are heeded*. HI children tend to be better at listening to them.

## *Participation in groups*

- *Participates with*: one other; small group; whole class.
- *Contributes*: on equal footing; mainly with reference to self; only if invited; not at all.
- *Adopts a role*: easily; reluctantly; will not attempt.

## Verbally mediated thinking

- *Classification*: colour; size; shape; collective nouns, etc.
- *Understands analogies and generalizations*
- *Pretending*: supposing; hypothesizing.

## Reading

It is anticipated that the school's usual record form, detailing various stages of attainment, will be used. The reading materials selected and the way in which they are presented are likely to be influenced by the information obtained in the preceding analysis.

## Writing

- *Gross motor skills*: A distinction should be made between enthusiastic and skilful. 'Good at football' often boils down to energetically chasing the ball. Many children with writing difficulties are clumsy and poorly coordinated. If there is poor control at this level, the fine movements required for quick, fluent writing cannot be made. When in doubt the school doctor should be asked to arrange for help to be given by the local Community Occupational or Physiotherapist, in the event of the locality having the good fortune to have one in post.
- *Fine motor skills*: Careful observation is called for in order to determine if fine hand control has developed. I see many children at second-

ary level (with normal hearing), who cannot easily move their fingers independently of each other, i.e. holding up the hand with fingers outstretched and bending each one at the middle joint sequentially. Many clumsy children have an intention tremor noticeable when they attempt any careful placement, be it bricks or a ruler on the paper, for drawing a straight line. The lack of coordination between the fingers on each hand and between both hands results in the children making a mess of things. Such children plump for Lego, since the pieces click into each other and exert the control that is lacking.

- *Pencil grip.*
- *Colouring*: keeping within the boundary.
- *Correct letter formation.*
- *Knowledge of letter names.*
- It needs to be remembered that with some they might only be identified correctly if the child can lip read. Even then additional clues might be called for, e.g. demonstrating in the air for maybe: s/t/z/j. Often when the spelling of a word has been asked the child will indicate when what is being said is not clear.
- *Spelling*:   Spelling needs to be taught quite specifically and in order not to miss out on anything a separate record should be kept detailing what has been covered. This would include the usual irregular words, normally included in spelling books. A note should be made of any words and families of words which are difficult for a hearing impaired child on account of the high frequency consonants. As already mentioned homophones (e.g. one/won; hue/hew; blue/blew, etc.) present their own peculiar difficulties as insufficient clues may have been derived from the context.

# Appendix II

# List of Useful Addresses

**The Royal National Institute for the Deaf**
Chief Executive: Mr. Michael Whitlam,
105 Gower Street, London WC1E 6AH.
Tel: 01-387 8033 (Voice) 01-387 6829 (Vistel)

**The Royal National Institute for the Deaf (Glasgow)**
Principal Officer: Mr C.J. Franchetti,
9 Clairmont Gardens,
Glasgow G3 7LW.
Tel: 041-332 0343

**The British Deaf Association**
Secretary General: Mr. A.W. Verney,
38 Victoria Place, Carlisle CA1 1HU.
Tel: Carlisle (0228) 48844 (Voice) and (0228) 28719 (Vistel/Minicom).
Telecom Gold: 79:BKUμ044. Prestel: 022 848 844

**The National Deaf Children's Society**
Director: Mr. H. Cayton,
45 Hereford Road, London W2 5AH.
Tel: 01-229 9272/4

**The National Deaf Children's Society**
Technology Information Centre,
Head of Centre: Mr. T. Winstanley,
4 Church Road, Edgbaston, Birmingham, B15 3TD.
Tel: (021) 454 5151 Voice. (021) 454 9795 Vistel.
Freefone 0800 424545. For parents only, between 1.00-5.00pm.

**The British Association of the Hard of Hearing**
Secretary General: Mr. Christopher Shaw,
7/11 Armstrong Road, London W3 7JL.
Tel: 01-745 1110/1353. Vistel: 01-743 1492

**The Sympathetic Hearing Scheme**
Co-ordinator: Marwood Braund,
7-11 Armstrong Road,
London W3 7JL.
Tel: 01-743 1492

**Breakthrough Trust Deaf-Hearing Integration**
National Director: Mr. David Hyslop,
Charles W. Gillett Centre,
Selly Oak Colleges, Birmingham B29 6LE.
Tel: 021-472 6447 (Voice) 021-471-1001 (Vistel)

**Network for the Handicapped**
(free legal and advisory service for disabled people and their families)
16 Princeton Street,
London WC1R 4BB.
Tel: 01-831 7740

# Glossary

## Acuity

Acuity is an indication of how well a signal can be detected. In respect of hearing acuity is good when very quiet sounds can be heard. For young adults the ability to hear sounds at 0 decibels represents good acuity (cf. **function**).

## Aids

### Body (worn)

High-powered aid. The mould is attached to a receiver (button), connected to the body of the aid by a lead.

### Ear level

Individual aid worn hooked over the pinna, with a close fitting mould. Children with a high frequency loss should have the shortest possible projection into the canal consistent with a good seal and a large channel through the middle. The amplification produced can range from low to near that of a body worn aid.

### Radio

The signal is transmitted on a radio frequency from the microphone (worn by the teacher) to the child's aid. This signal can be disrupted by illegal use of the same frequency. In the event of more than one child using such an aid in the same school arrangements have to be made to ensure different frequencies are used in different settings.

*Type I*  A body-worn aid picks up the signal.

*Type II*  The receiver is connected to the child's own ear-level aid. The argument for this type of aid is that a more consistent sound pattern is received by the child. Different aids (even of the same make) have varying tonal characteristics.

## Settings

ON/OFF/T: With the switch in the ON position the microphone in the aid is functional. A drawback is the amount of ambient noise picked up, which can mask speech. The 'T' position only allows the sound picked up by the transmitting microphone (usually very close to the speaker) to be received. Some of the most sophisticated systems permit the microphone on the aid to function at the same time as the 'T' setting.

## Ambient noise

All the varied sounds in the environment. These include *impact* noises, as when a book is slapped down on a desk.

## Acupaedia

A method of teaching children with severe/profound hearing losses in which the child is taught solely through use of residual hearing.

## Audiometer

A calibrated instrument for measuring the loudness at which pure tones can be detected. Pure tones are sounds consisting of only one frequency.

## Clinically normal

### Hearing within normal limits (HWNL)

The ability to detect pure tones at 25 decibels or less for each of the frequencies tested is said to indicate hearing is clinically normal.

## Cochlear implant

A surgical procedure whereby an electrode is threaded into the cochlear. There is a subcutaneous receiver that picks up signals from the hearing aid, worn externally.

# Cued speech

A system of hand and finger movements devised to indicate which of one or more sounds are being made, when the visual pattern is the same, e.g. d/t; k/g. Every sound has an accompanying hand configuration and/or movement.

# Decibel

A measurement of loudness, 0 db being the quietest sound that can just be heard by a young adult with normal hearing.

# Ear

## *Cochlear*

The complex organ that receives mechanical stimulation conveyed via the middle ear by the ossicles, which have been set in motion by sound waves striking the ear drum. It analyses the frequency of the waves and transforms movement into electrical impulses, which travel up the auditory nerve to the brain.
*Ossicles* (little bones) – *malleus, incus* and *stapes* – *located in the middle ear.*

## *Stapedius*

The muscle with the highest nerve to muscle fibre ratio in the body that can influence the movements of the ossicles in such a way as to enhance detection of high frequency sounds – especially unvoiced consonants. It is located in the middle ear.

## *Tensor tympani*

The other muscle in the middle ear. It complements the action of the stapedius. It can stiffen the ear-drum so it is more sensitive to high frequency sounds. It is also powerful enough to vibrate the drum.

## *Tympanum*

Ear-drum, hence *tympanoplasty* – plastic surgery to repair diseased and damaged drums.

## Eustachian tube

A tube connecting the back of the throat to the middle ear. When healthy air can pass up and down freely to keep the air pressure in the middle ear at atmospheric pressure. It is more likely to become blocked and infected in young children due to the angle. As we grow older the elongation of the face increases the slope and assists drainage.

## False positive

This is a result that suggests the condition is present when it is not. A false positive is most likely to be obtained by the inexperienced clinician.

## Frequency

Sounds can be described in terms of frequency (herz (Hz) and Kiloherz (KHz)). Middle C on the piano is approximately 250 Hz. Each speech sound has one or more characteristic frequency. As herz refers to events that occur in one second, cps (cycles per second) and herz are used interchangeably, e.g. 500 cps or 500 hz. Herz was the person who originated such definitions.

## Function

Function relates to the quality of performance. An older person may not be able to hear as well as a younger person yet still be able to make more efficient use of what is heard.

## Glue ear (OM)

### *Terminology*

(*Otitis media*)

| | |
|---|---|
| Serous OM | Suppurative OM |
| Secretory OM | Bacterial OM |
| Mucoid OM | Purulent |
| Non-suppurative OM | |

*Acute:* 1–6 weeks, *Subacute:* 6–9 weeks, *Chronic:* 12+ weeks.

*Manifestation*

| Painless | Painful |
| Silent | Screaming |
| Insidious | Sudden onset |
| Sterile | Infected |

*Treatment*

Antihistamine            Antibiotic
Decongestant

Remove tonsils and adenoids myringotomy and grommet insertion.
*Note*: There are differences of opinion concerning the efficacy of treatment of glue ear.

## Grommets and T-Tubes

Grommets are like little hollow spindles, pushed through the ear-drum, after any secretions have been removed, to allow air into the middle ear. T–Tubes are slightly larger and used when the problem is persistent.

## Habituation

The psychological process whereby an irrelevant (to the individual concerned) stimulus is ignored if repeated frequently. It occurs to both auditory and visual stimuli in particular, making distracting noises and uninteresting sights fade into the background.

## Hearing impairment (loss)

*Causes*

CONGENITAL

Existing at birth. It may be genetically determined or the result of infection, e.g. rubella. Drugs of various kinds taken during pregnancy can also be a cause.

ACQUIRED OR ADVENTITIOUS

This can result from infections, trauma and certain categories of drugs, e.g. some antibiotics.

PRESBYCUSIS

The gradual hearing loss, especially in the high frequencies that accompanies ageing.

## Degree

There are complex criteria for categorising the degree of hearing loss. Those given below must be regarded as rule of thumb.

| *Mild* | *Moderate* | *Severe* | *Profound* |
|---|---|---|---|
| Up to 35 dbs | 35–55 dbs | 55–75+ dbs | 75+ – no response to sound |

## Types

CONDUCTIVE

Any condition that impedes sound passing through the air reaching the inner ear normally. The most common causes are: *glue ear* (otitis media – see above); *oto-sclerosis* (abnormal growth of the bone that fuses the stapes into the oval window); *meatal atresia* (the canal is absent or very tiny) – the pinna is often absent or rudimentary; *abnormalities* of the ossicular chain (the three little bones in the middle ear); perforated ear-drums.

SENSORI-NEURAL

*Peripheral*: Damage or abnormality of the nerves in the inner ear.
*Central*: Damage or abnormalities at any site in the auditory pathways or projection areas of the cortex. *Aphasics* are often able to detect sounds normally but they cannot make sense of what they hear. In other respects they appear to be of normal intelligence.

MIXED

This is caused by a sensori-neural loss with a conductive overlay. The sensori-neural component is incurable. The conductive element is often amenable to treatment.

## Impendance bridge (middle-ear analyser)

An instrument for checking the function of the middle ear, the movement of the drum, ossicles and the stapedial reflex.

# Kinaesthetic

Pertaining to the information fed back to the brain from the receptors in the muscles in the limbs and body, when a movement is made. Some of the receptors are coordinated with the semicircular canals and provide ongoing information about posture.

# Oto-acoustic emissions

The ear is not a passive receiver, simply responding to sound waves. The ear produces sounds that can be detected by placing a small sensitive microphone in the canal. This means the muscles in the middle ear vibrate the drum sufficiently to make detectable sounds. These sounds are always absent when there is a conductive hearing loss. This suggests a possible reason for the sometimes inordinate affect on auditory discrimination of quite small losses in acuity. The necessary interaction between the sounds made by the ears, facilitating discrimination is prevented.

# Personality traits

## *Endogenous*

These are traits such as introversion and extroversion, which appear to be largely genetically determined.

## *Exogenous*

This refers to external circumstances to which we react. It encompasses socio-economic and child rearing factors as well as day to day events which have an effect on the way we feel and behave.

# Proprioceptive

Relating to sensations derived from any part of the body that are not related specifically to movement, e.g. pressure; temperature, auditory feedback from own speech inside the head (i.e. through bone-conduction).

# Sound

Sound can be analysed according to loudness (measured in decibels) and pitch (measured in cycles per second – often referred to as Herz).

## Tests

### Distraction

The child is settled quietly or engaged by an assistant in some quiet occupation. Sounds are made outside the child's field of vision. An indication that the sound has been heard may be turning of the head and trunk, swivelling of the eyes or as little as stilling. Very careful observation is called for in some cases, *habituation* can occur if the same sounds are repeated too frequently giving a *false positive*. Distraction tests are used in the age range 7 months–2$^1$/2 years or when there is evidence of mental retardation.

### Performance

- Free field
  The child is required to perform some action, e.g. place one stacking beaker inside another; put a peg in a board, when a sound is heard.
- Closed circuit
  The child wears headphones to listen to pure tones made by a carefully calibrated audiometer. The responses may be the same as for the free-field condition, pressing a switch or saying yes. Occasionally a child will not respond at threshold and an instruction to say when the sound has not been heard elicits a response whenever the sounds are heard. This is usually symptomatic of emotional disturbance. Occasionally it is simply an excuse to have time off school.
  The *Sweep Test* is simply a closed circuit test carried out in schools to check whether the child can hear across the range of frequencies at 25 decibels in both ears.

### Impedance

This is a check of middle ear function and is used to check on information that may be obtained by a visual inspection of the drum with an *otoscope*. It does at times detect abnormalities that may not be perceived by such means.

### ERA (brain stem)

To obtain an *evoked response audiogram* electrodes are attached to the head. The patterns of waves can be interpreted to see if sounds have been detected. With young children they have to be given medication to make them drowsy. As other types of test are more useful the ERA is only used when for some reason other methods cannot be used, e.g. the child is exceptionally overactive or uncooperative.

## *Speech tests*

- *Motor response*
  Read Picture Test: A series of cards. The child has to point to the appropriate picture.
  Kendall Toy Test: The child selects the toy object named.
  McCormick Test: The child selects the toy named.
- Verbal response.
  A.B. Word Lists
  Manchester Junior Word List
  The examiner reads a list of words consisting of three phonemes (CVC – e.g. sh'i'p) one at a time. The child repeats each word. Any errors are scored (3 – all correct; 0 – none correct)
  Lists can be read under different conditions, i.e. with or without lip reading; with or without aid; at different loudness levels; at different distances from the speaker. In this way a *speech audiogram* may be obtained. Properly interpreted this could be used to provide information about how well the child is able to function under varying classroom conditions.

To date no one has succeeded in devising a satisfactory test for the discrimination of continuous speech. Apologists claim single words are more difficult to discriminate because of the lack of context, so nothing much would be gained from a more extended analysis. A classroom teacher who had been told a child only has a very mild loss which should not be of any significance might well question such a statement in the light of experience.

## Total communication

A teaching method in which, in addition to teaching the children to speak and lip read, signs and finger spelling are used as adjuncts. There might also be greater emphasis on the use of touch, movement, etc. as well. (See Chapter 6 on writing especially and Appendix A, Historical Perspectives.)

## Vibrotactile

When sounds, especially low ones, are made very loud they stimulate touch receptors. They can be felt by leaning over the speaker of a public address system or touching the sounding board of a piano. Profoundly hearing impaired children can be helped to detect sound by holding a vibrator, activated by a kind of hearing aid.

# References and Further Reading

AMON, C. (1988). *'Remediation within and beyond state and federal guidelines'* (pp. 149-155), in *Auditory Disorders in School Children*, (2nd ed), Roeser, R.J. and Downs, M.P. (eds and contributors), New York: Thieme Medical Publishers Inc.

BARHAM, I. (1987). 'Mathematics for the deaf child', *Soundbarrier, the Journal of the RNID* (Including BTA Newsletter), 14, pp. 14-15.

BESS, F.H., FREEMAN, B.A. and SINCLAIR, J.S. (eds) (1981). *Amplification in Education*, Alexander Graham Bell Association for the Deaf, 3417 Volta Place N.W., Washington DC 20007.

BONNET, J.P. (1620). *Simplification of the Letters of the Alphabet and Method of Teaching Deaf Mutes to Speak*. Madrid: Francisco.

BRUNER, J.S. (1960). *The Process of Education*. New York: Vintage Books/Alfred Knopf/Random House.

DE L'EPEE, C.M. (1789). *The True Manner of Instructing the Deaf and Dumb, confirmed by Long Experience*. Paris: Chez Nyon L'Aine.

FLAVELL, J.H. (1963). *The Developmental Psychology of Jean Piaget*. New York: Van Nostrand.

FURTH, H.G. (1966). *Thinking Without Language*, Free Press, New York.

KEINER, R. (1981). *Music for Deaf Children: a practical guide for teachers and parents*, London: The author (copy in RNID Library).

KRUTETSKI, V.A. (Tr. Joan Teller) (1976). *The Psychology of Mathematical Abilities in Schoolchildren*. University of Chicago, Chicago, Ill.

MCCORMICK, B. (1988). *Screening for Hearing Impairment in Young Children*. London: Croom Helm.

MOORES, D.F. (1978). *Educating the Deaf. Psychology, Principles and Practices*. Houghton Mifflin Company, Boston, Mass.

O'CONNOR, N. and HERMELIN, B. (1972). 'Seeing and hearing in space and time'. *Perception and Psychophysics*. 11, pp. 46–8.

ROBBINS, C. and ROBBINS, C. (1980). *A Resource Manual and Curriculum Guide*. Audiological Introduction by Arthur Boothroyd, Magnamusic, Baton, Rouge.

SCOUTEN, E.L. (1984). *Turning Points in the Education of Deaf People*. Danville, Illinois: The Interstate Printers and Publishers.

STOKOE, W., CRONEBERG, C. and CASTERLINE, D. *A Dictionary of American Sign Language*. Washington DC, Gallaudet College 1965. 2nd ed (1976). STOKOE, W.C. Linstok Press.

VERNON, M. (1967). 'Relationship of Language to the Thinking Process'. *Archives of General Psychiatry*. 16, pp. 325–33.

**National Curriculum Documents** (All available free from the Department of Education and Science and the Welsh Office):

Task Group on Assessment and Testing (TGAT). A Report, December 1987.

Design and Technology Working Group. Interim Report, November 1988.

English for ages 5 to 11. Proposals of the Secretary of State for Education and Science and the Secretary of State for Wales, November 1988.

Mathematics for ages 5 to 16. Proposals of the Secretary of State for Education and Science and the Secretary of State for Wales, August 1988.

Science for ages 5 to 6. Proposals of the Secretary of State for Education and Science and the Secretary of State for Wales, August 1988.

## Books used in Schools for the Deaf and in Partially Hearing Units

*Bangers and Mash*, Longmans.

*Big Books* (Mathematics), Ginn.

*Domino Picture Books*, Oliver and Boyd.

*Flightpath to Reading*, Sheila McCullagh, E.J. Arnold.

*Frog Books*, Mercer Mayer. Collins.
*Graded Reader*, Oxford University Press.
*Help*, Nelson.
*Mike and Mandy*, Nelson.
*Mirror Books*, Andre Deutsch.
*Music for Children.* (3 vols), Orff Schulwerk Schott, American Edition.
*Music Time*, Teacher's Book. BBC.
*Nuffield Maths.*
*\*Once Upon a Time* series. Ginn.
*One, Two, Three and Away*, Rupert Hart Davis.
*Science for Children with Learning Difficulties*, Macdonald.
*Scottish Primary Mathematics Group*, Heinemann.
*\*Simplified Stories*, Ginn.
*\*Sparks Readers*, Blackie. Granada Publishing Hart Educational.
*Stories in Pictures.* John Goodall Macmillan.
*Story Chest.* Arnold Wheaton Pergamon Press.
*\*The Berry House Books*, Wheaton.
*The Oxford Reading Tree.* Oxford University Press.
*Topsy and Sam.* Cassell and Co.
*Trog Books.* Methuen Educational.
*Titles marked with an asterisk are of particular interest to teachers.

# Equipment used in Schools for the Deaf and PHUs

*Fizzog.* Galt Toys.
*Harlequin coloured cubes.* Philograph publications.
*Sequence and Rhythm boards.* Philograph publications.
*Symmetry and reversal pairing cards.* Philograph.

# PRACTICAL INTEGRATION IN EDUCATION

A new series of books focusing on the practical aspects of integrating
children with special needs into mainstream schools.
Each book focuses on a particular handicap and will provide you with:

- Relevant factual information about the handicap

- Suggestions for overcoming problems

- Methods of helping these children to integrate

- Practical tips on aids, equipment, classroom design and career advice

Following the 1981 Education Act pupils who would formerly have
attended special schools were integrated into ordinary schools. The Practical
Integration in Education series investigates the problems of integration
experienced by pupils and their teachers. The series puts forward a number
of suggestions of ways in which successful integration may be facilitated
making it an invaluable addition to any teachers bookshelf.

**Partially Sighted Children** is the first in the series and brings together a
wide range of knowledge and experience about the educational needs of
children with partial sight to enable mainstream teachers and nursery
teachers to cater for the needs of visually impaired children in their
classroom. It draws on information gained through experience and research
on aspects such as special equipment needs, classroom design, mobility
problems and their solution – including a chapter devoted to sport and
leisure activities – and the future career prospects open
to partially sighted students.

The authors, Gianetta Corley, Steve Lockett and Donald Robinson, are all
experts in the field of visual impairment and the book benefits from their
breadth of experience and different perspectives. Donald Robinson who has
retired as Head of a school for the visually impaired, spent his career
teaching blind and partially sighted children; Steve Lockett works as a
Mobility Teacher and Gianetta Corley is an Educational Psychologist for
visually impaired children.

ISBN 07005 1198 0  Code 8311 021 – Price £6.95

Coming soon:
**The Motor Impaired Child**
Myra Tingle

For further information, please contact our
Customer Support Department on (0753) 858961,
or write to the following address:

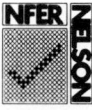

NFER-NELSON, Darville House,
2 Oxford Road East, Windsor,
Berkshire SL4 1DF